99 Detox Smoothies for Weight Loss

The Path to Vibrancy

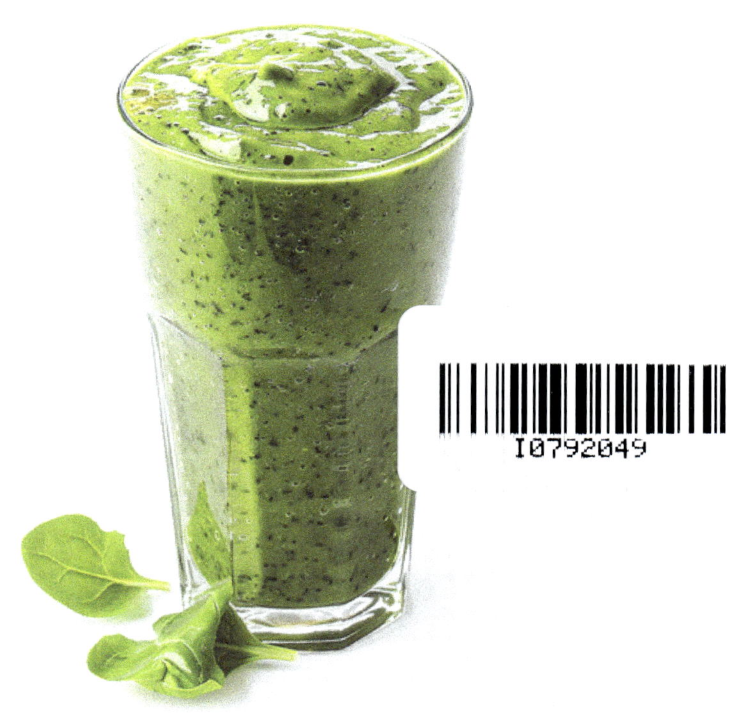

Olivia Klein © 2024

Intro

Welcome to a journey that promises not just transformation but a vibrant renewal of your body and spirit. "Detox Smoothies for Weight Loss" is more than a book; it's a gateway to a healthier, more vibrant you. In the pages that follow, you will discover the power of whole foods blended into deliciously potent smoothies, each designed to cleanse your body, boost your metabolism, and shed unwanted pounds.

In a world where processed foods and artificial ingredients dominate our diets, causing harm to our bodies and clouding our minds, the need for a reset button is more pressing than ever. This book offers just that—a natural way to detoxify your body, reclaim your energy, and set the foundation for long-term health and weight management.

But this is not just about losing weight. It's about finding a balance. It's about nourishing your body with essential nutrients, vitamins, and minerals through the simplest and most basic of human traditions: eating real, whole foods. Our smoothies are crafted from fruits, vegetables, nuts, seeds, and herbs—each ingredient selected for its nutritional benefits and detoxifying properties.

As you turn these pages, you'll learn not only how to create these delicious beverages but also understand why they work. You'll explore the science behind detoxification, how specific ingredients can support your body's natural detox pathways, and why blending these elements can maximize their nutritional impact.

"Detox Smoothies for Weight Loss" is designed to be your companion in creating a healthier lifestyle. Whether you're looking to jumpstart your weight loss journey, seeking to cleanse your body of toxins, or simply wishing to incorporate more fruits and vegetables into your diet, these smoothies offer a path toward achieving your goals.

Embrace the journey of transformation. Let each smoothie be a step toward a lighter, healthier, more vibrant you. Here's to your health, to your weight loss, and to a new way of living. Welcome to the beginning of your transformation.

Ingredients

1 cup spinach, 1 apple, 1 banana, 1 tablespoon chia seeds, 1 cup unsweetened almond milk

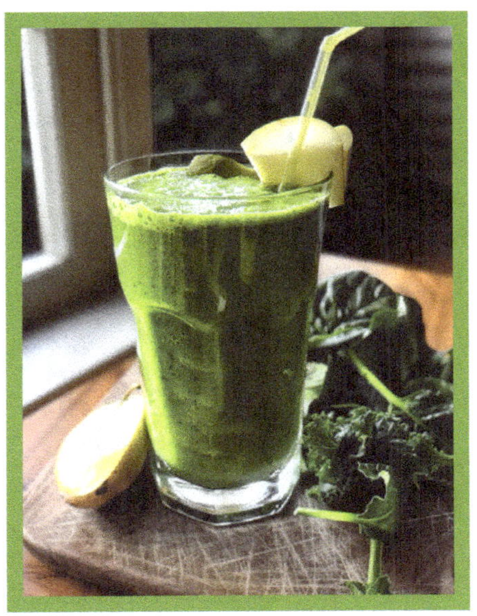

Benefits

Spinach is rich in iron and magnesium for energy production.

Ginger Zest Smoothie

Ingredients

1 cup kale, 1/2 cucumber, 1 lemon (juiced), 1 tablespoon grated ginger, 1 cup coconut water

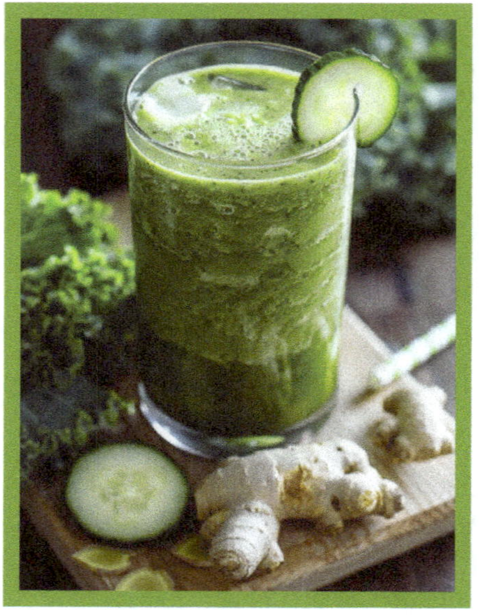

Benefits

Ginger has anti-inflammatory properties.

Berry Antioxidant Smoothie

Ingredients

1 cup mixed berries, 1 banana, 1 tablespoon flaxseeds,
1 cup Greek yogurt

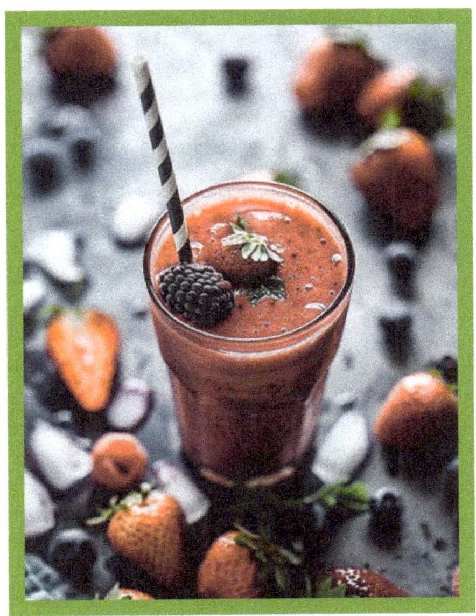

Benefits

Berries are high in antioxidants for fighting

inflammation.

Tropical Detox Smoothie

Ingredients

1 cup pineapple, 1/2 mango, 1/2 avocado, 1 teaspoon turmeric, 1 cup coconut water

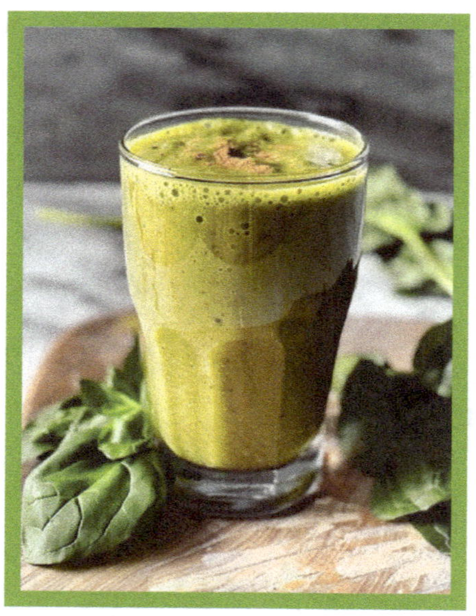

Benefits

Turmeric has powerful antioxidant effects.

Beetroot and Berry Flush

Ingredients

1 small beetroot, 1 cup frozen mixed berries, 1/2 lemon (juiced), 1 tablespoon chia seeds, 1 cup water

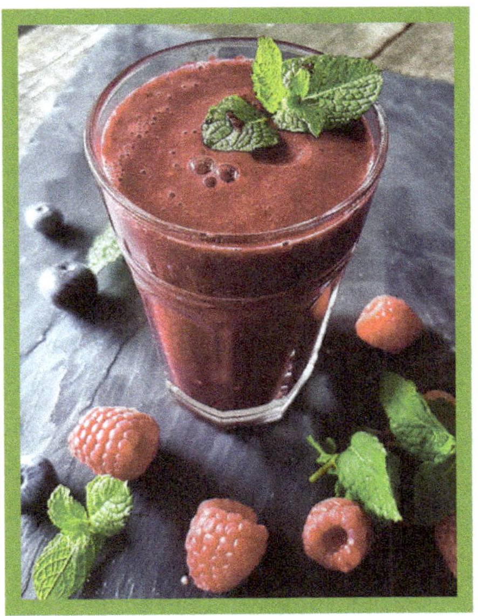

Benefits

Beetroot can help lower blood pressure.

Ingredients

1 cup brewed green tea, 1 cup spinach, 1 orange, 1/2 banana, 1 tablespoon honey

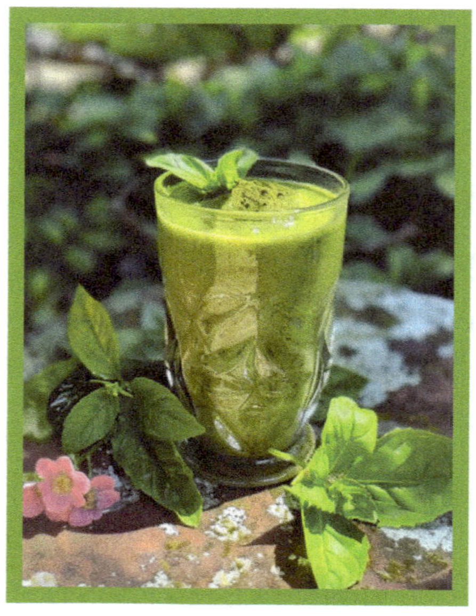

Benefits

Green tea boosts metabolism with its catechins content.

Ingredients

1 apple, 1 banana, 1/2 teaspoon cinnamon, 1 tablespoon ground flaxseed, 1 cup unsweetened almond milk

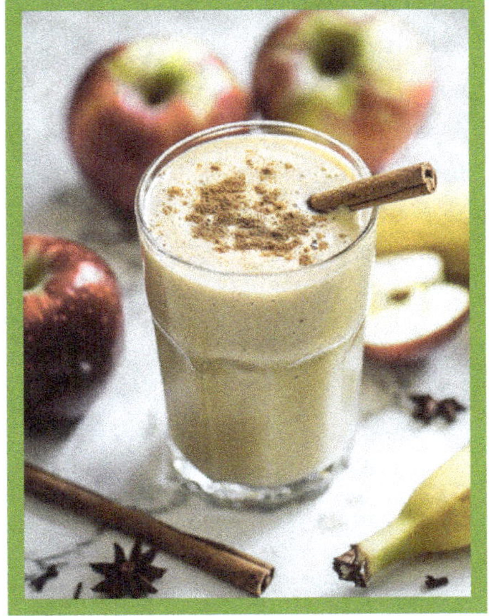

Benefits

Cinnamon helps regulate blood sugar levels.

Carrot Ginger Cleanse

Ingredients

2 carrots, 1 apple, 1 tablespoon grated ginger, 1/2 lemon (juiced), 1 cup water

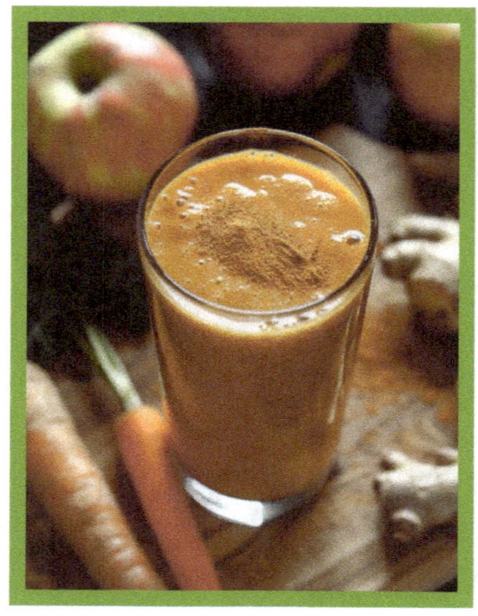

Benefits

Carrots are rich in vitamin A and beta-carotene.

Spicy Avocado Smoothie

Ingredients

1/2 avocado, 1 cup spinach, 1/2 cucumber, 1/2 jalapeño, 1 cup water

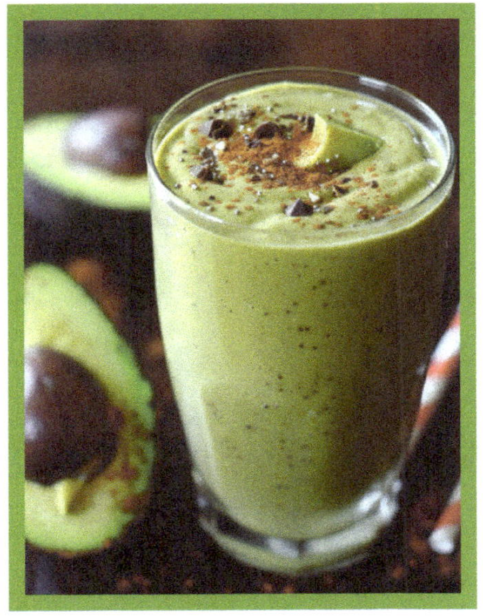

Benefits

Avocado is high in healthy fats and fiber.

Cucumber Mint Refresh

Ingredients

1 cucumber, 1/2 cup mint leaves, 1/2 lemon (juiced), 1 tablespoon honey, 1 cup water

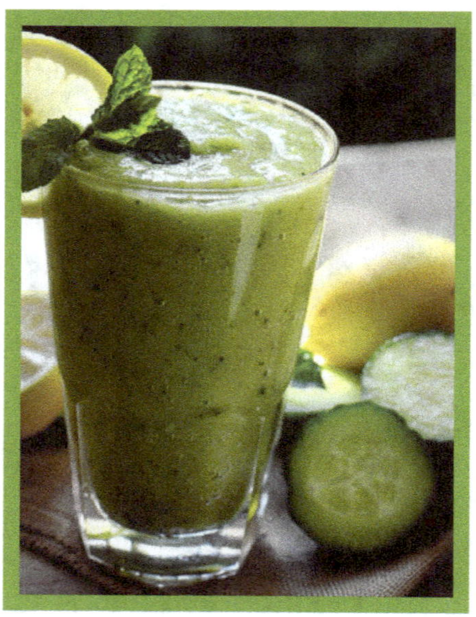

Benefits

Mint aids in digestion and inflammation.

Pineapple Spinach Flush

Ingredients

1 cup pineapple chunks, 1 cup spinach, 1/2 cucumber, 1 tablespoon flax seeds, 1 cup water

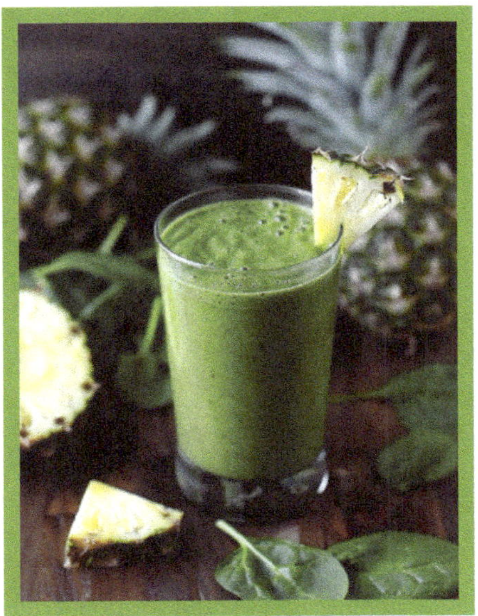

Benefits

Pineapple contains bromelain, which aids in digestion.

Citrus Beet Cleanser

Ingredients

1 small beet, 1 orange, 1/2 grapefruit, 1/2 lemon (juiced), 1 inch ginger, 1 cup water

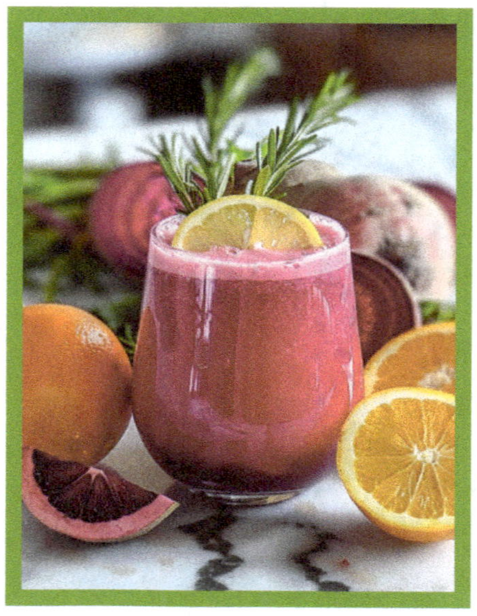

Benefits

Beets help detoxify the liver and purify the blood.

Watermelon Mint Detox

Ingredients

2 cups cubed watermelon, 1/2 cup mint leaves, 1 lime (juiced), 1 cup coconut water

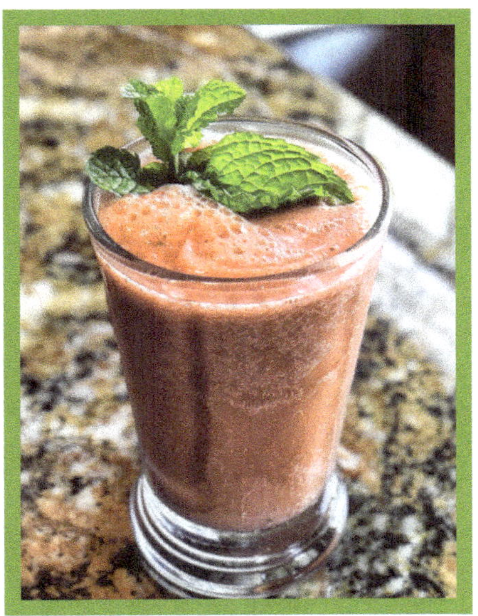

Benefits

Watermelon is hydrating and helps flush out toxins.

Ingredients

1 avocado, juice of 2 limes, 1 cup spinach, 1 tablespoon chia seeds, 1 cup almond milk

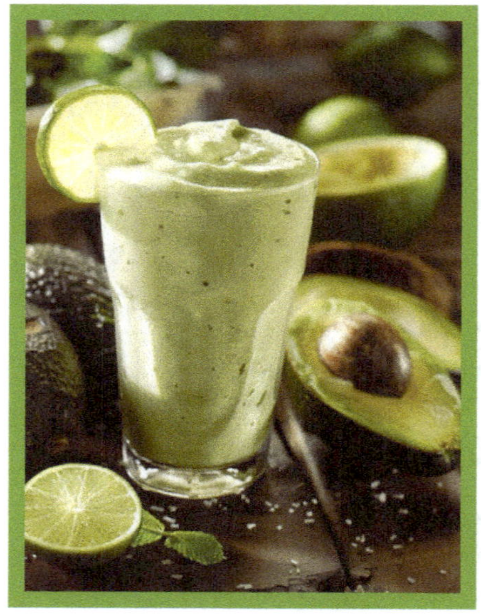

Benefits

Avocado provides healthy fats that keep you satiated.

Blueberry Lemonade Bliss

Ingredients

1 cup blueberries, juice of 1 lemon, 1 tablespoon raw honey, 1 cup water, 1 teaspoon spirulina

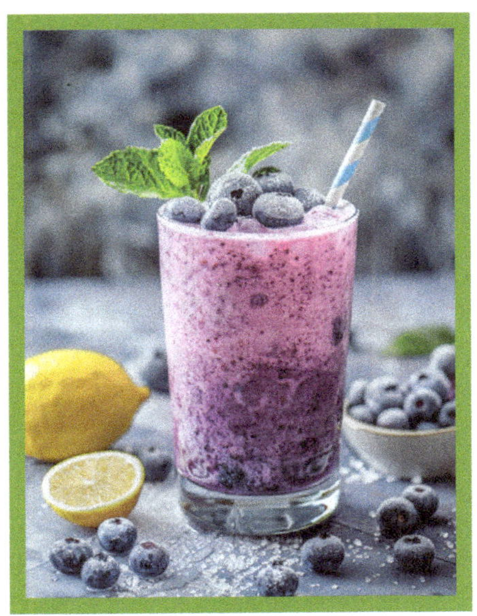

Benefits

Blueberries are high in antioxidants.

Spicy Pineapple Turmeric Kick

Ingredients

1 cup pineapple chunks, 1 teaspoon turmeric, 1/2 teaspoon cayenne pepper, 1 cup coconut water

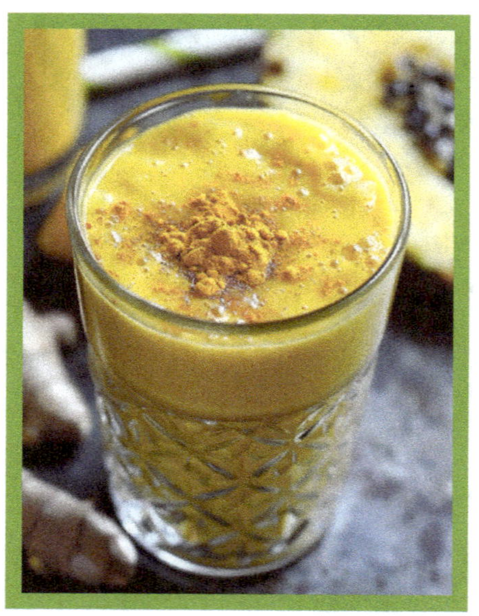

Benefits

Turmeric and cayenne pepper boost metabolism.

Kale Ginger Glow

Ingredients

1 cup kale, 1 inch ginger, 1 pear, 1 apple, 1 cup water

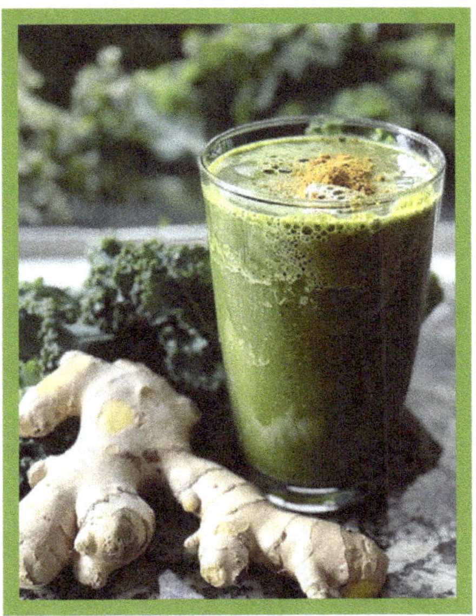

Benefits

Kale is nutrient-dense and supports healthy skin.

Carrot Apple Zing

Ingredients

2 carrots, 1 apple, 1/2 lemon (juiced), 1 inch ginger, 1 cup water

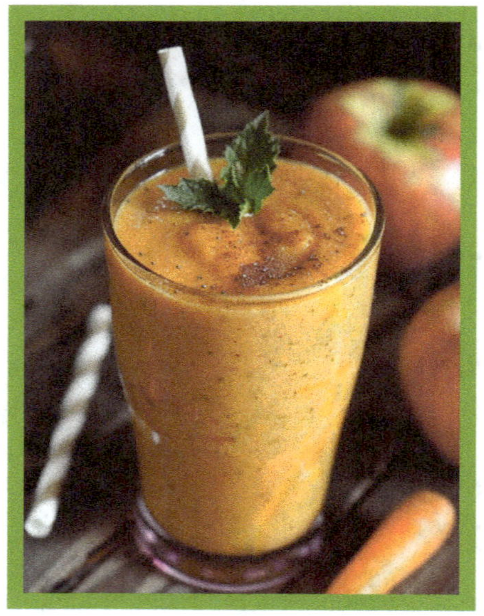

Benefits

Carrots are rich in beta-carotene for eye health.

Cucumber Kiwi Quench

Ingredients

1 cucumber, 2 kiwis, 1/2 cup parsley, 1/2 lemon (juiced), 1 cup water

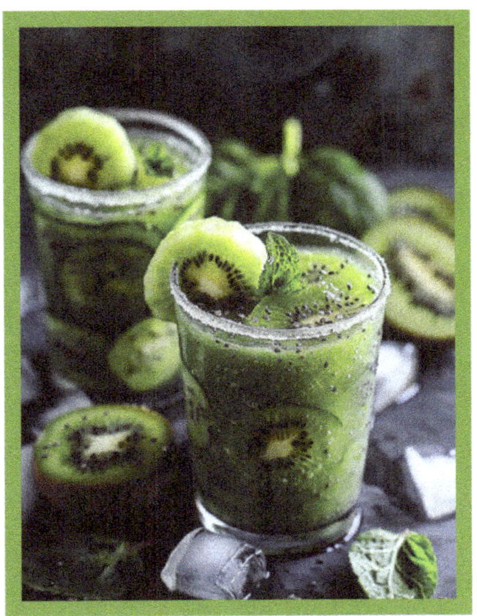

Benefits

Kiwi is rich in vitamin C and dietary fiber.

Raspberry Lime Refresher

Ingredients

1 cup raspberries, juice of 2 limes, 1 tablespoon flax seeds, 1 cup water

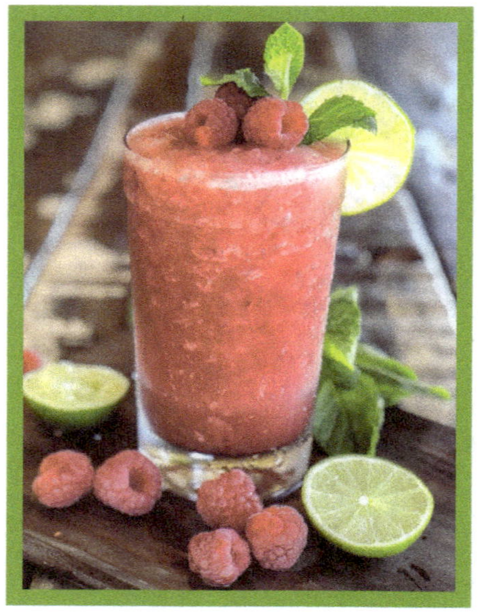

Benefits

Raspberries are high in fiber and vitamins.

Ingredients

1 banana, 1 tsp spirulina powder, 1 cup spinach, 1/2 avocado, 1 cup almond milk

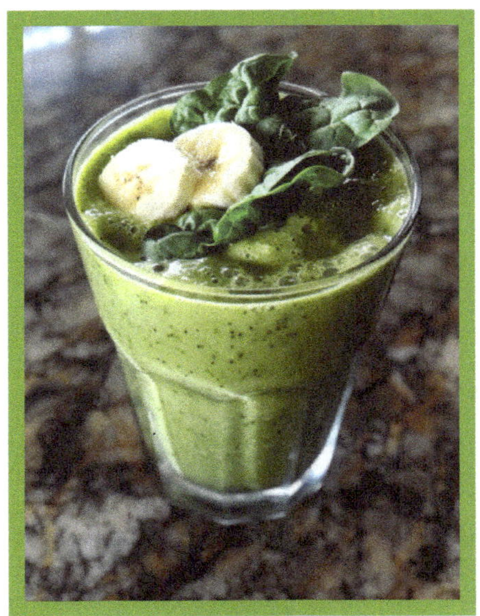

Benefits

Spirulina is a superfood rich in protein and vitamins.

Golden Ginger Smoothie

Ingredients

1 cup mango chunks, 1/2 tsp turmeric, 1 inch ginger, 1/2 lemon, 1 cup coconut water

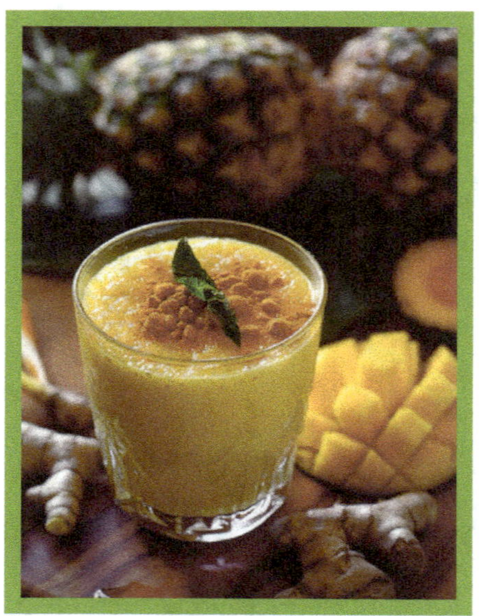

Benefits

Turmeric has anti-inflammatory properties.

Coco-Berry Detox

Ingredients

1 cup strawberries, 1/2 cup raspberries, 1 cup coconut water, 1 tbsp flaxseed

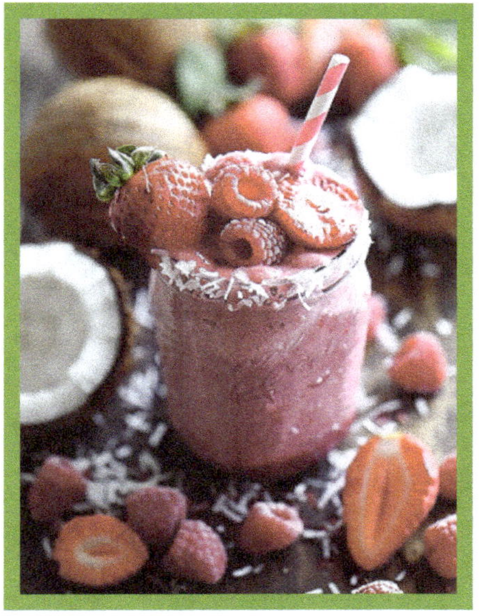

Benefits

Berries are loaded with antioxidants.

Pep in Your Step

Ingredients

1/2 cup kale, 1/2 cup parsley, 1 apple, 1/2 lemon, 1 inch ginger, 1 cup water

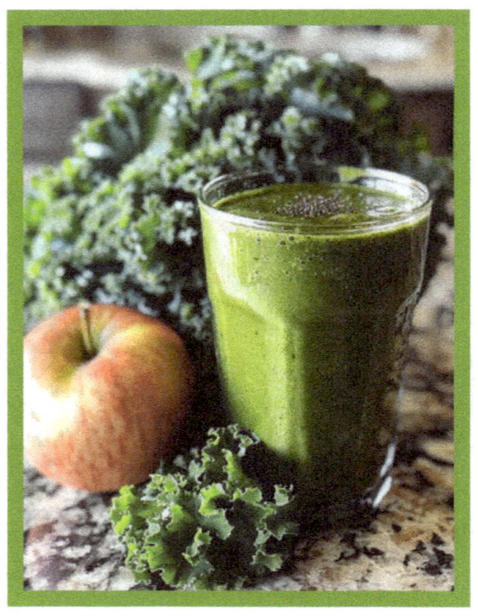

Benefits

Parsley is a natural diuretic to reduce bloating.

Ingredients

1 small beet, 1 carrot, 1 orange, 1/2 inch ginger, 1 cup water

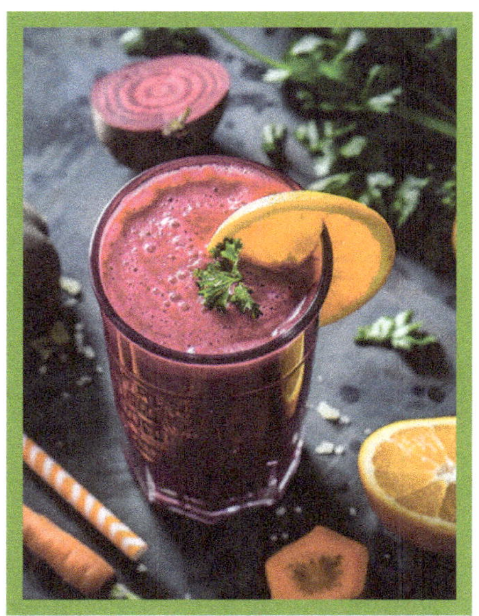

Benefits

Beetroot can increase stamina and exercise performance.

Tropical Turmeric Cleanser

Ingredients

1/2 cup pineapple, 1/2 cup mango, 1/2 tsp turmeric, 1/2 lemon, 1 cup orange juice

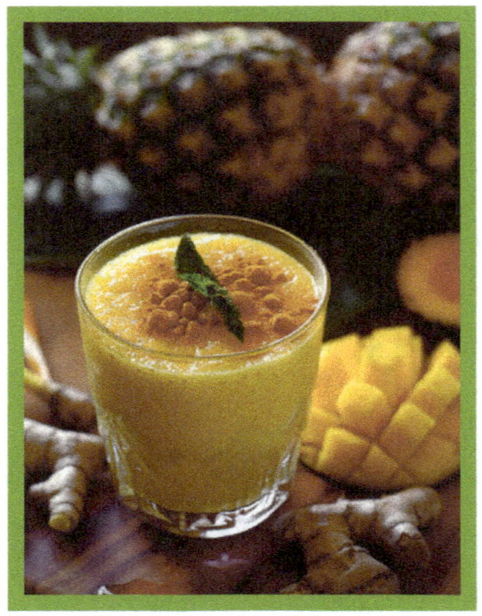

Benefits

Pineapple aids digestion and boosts immunity.

Ingredients

1 cup brewed green tea (cooled), 1 cup spinach, 1/2 apple, juice of 1 lime

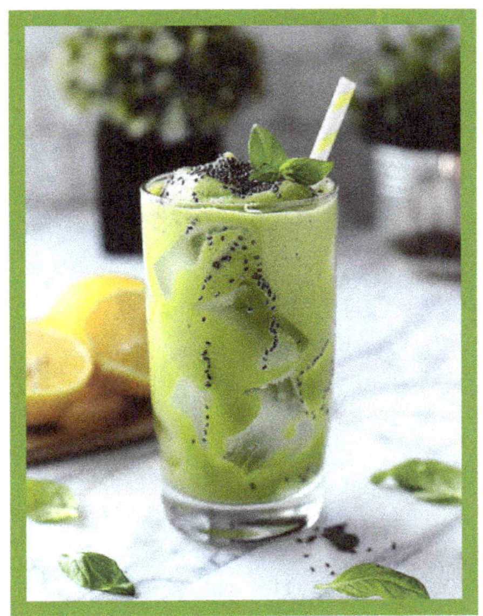

Benefits

Green tea boosts metabolism and burns fat.

Ingredients

1 large cucumber, 1/2 cup mint leaves, juice of 1 lime, 1 tbsp honey, 1 cup water

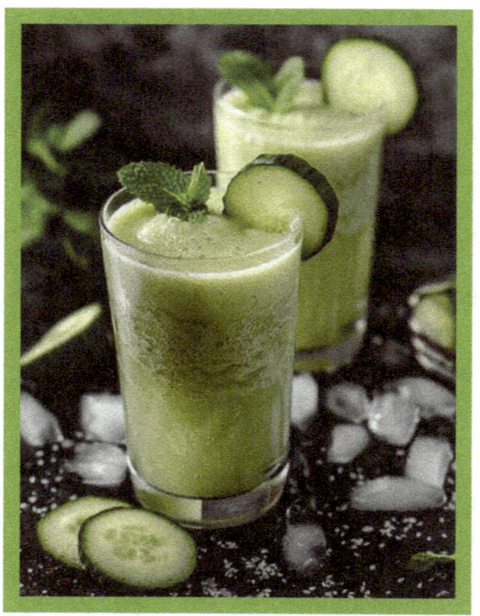

Benefits

Cucumber is hydrating and supports skin health.

Sweet Potato Pie Smoothie

Ingredients

1/2 cooked sweet potato, 1/2 banana, 1 tsp cinnamon, 1 cup almond milk, 1 tbsp maple syrup

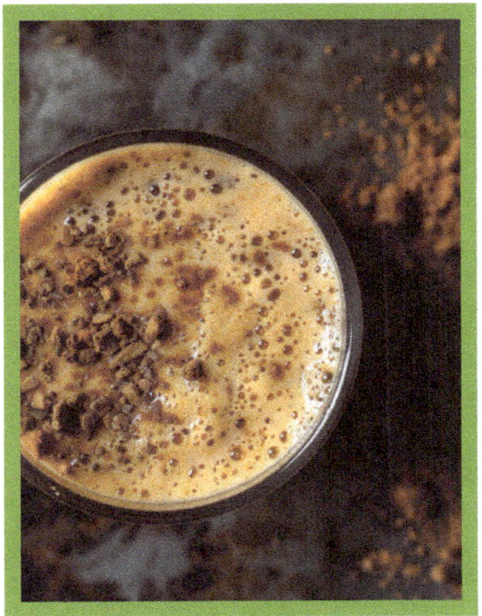

Benefits

Sweet potatoes are high in fiber and vitamins.

Chia Berry Flush

Ingredients

1 cup mixed berries, 1 tbsp chia seeds, 1 cup spinach, 1 cup coconut water

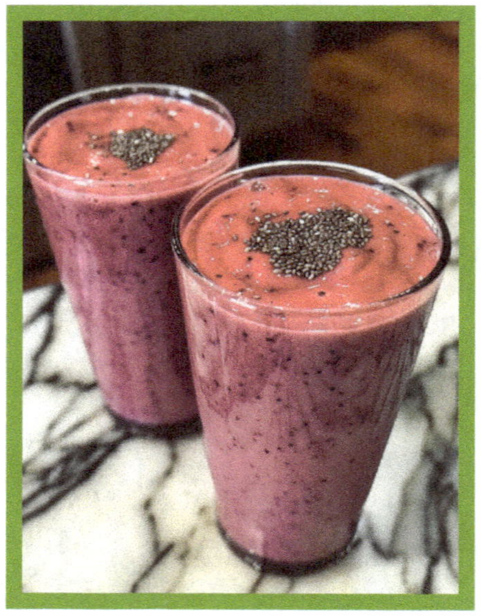

Benefits

Chia seeds are rich in omega-3 fatty acids and fiber.

Avocado Green Tea Smoothie

Ingredients

1/2 ripe avocado, 1 cup strong brewed green tea (cooled), 1/2 banana, 1 cup spinach, 1 tsp honey

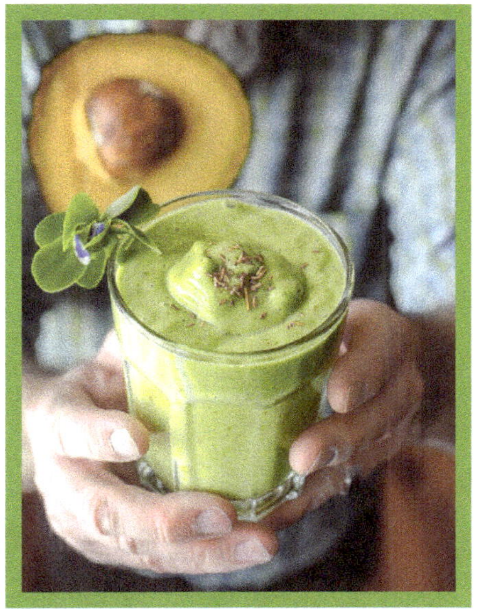

Benefits

Green tea is renowned for its metabolism-boosting properties.

Berry Ginger Blast

Ingredients

1 cup mixed berries (strawberries, blueberries, raspberries), 1 inch fresh ginger, 1 cup almond milk, 1 tbsp chia seeds

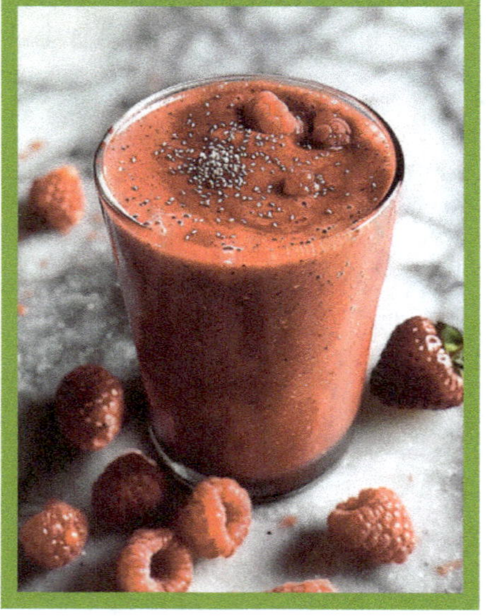

Benefits

Ginger can help soothe digestion and reduce inflammation.

Ingredients

1 orange, 1/2 grapefruit, 1/2 lemon (juiced), 1 cup kale, 1 tsp flaxseed oil, 1 cup water

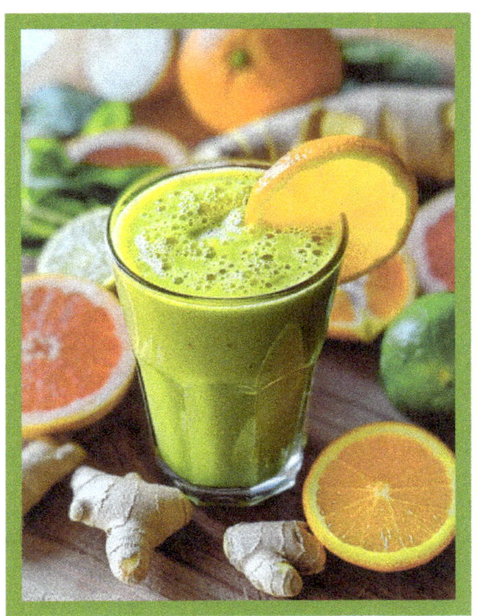

Benefits

Citrus fruits are high in Vitamin C, boosting the immune system.

Ingredients

1 large cucumber, 1/2 cup fresh mint leaves, 1 lime (juiced), 1/2 green apple, 1 cup water

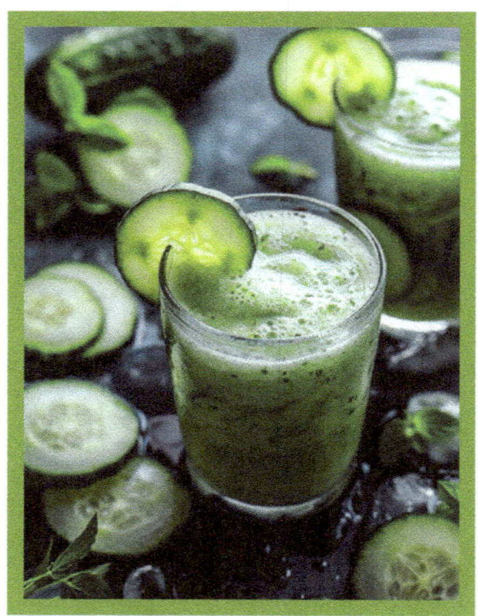

Benefits

Cucumber provides hydration and essential vitamins.

Ingredients

1/2 cup beetroot, 1 carrot, 1 apple, 1/2 inch turmeric root, 1 cup water, 1 tbsp lemon juice

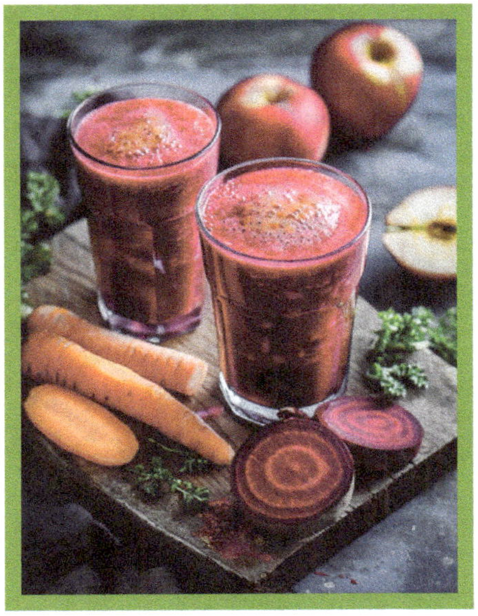

Benefits

Beetroot detoxifies the liver and purifies the blood.

Mango Spinach Glow

Ingredients

1 cup mango chunks, 1 cup spinach, 1/2 avocado, 1/2 lemon (juiced), 1 cup coconut water

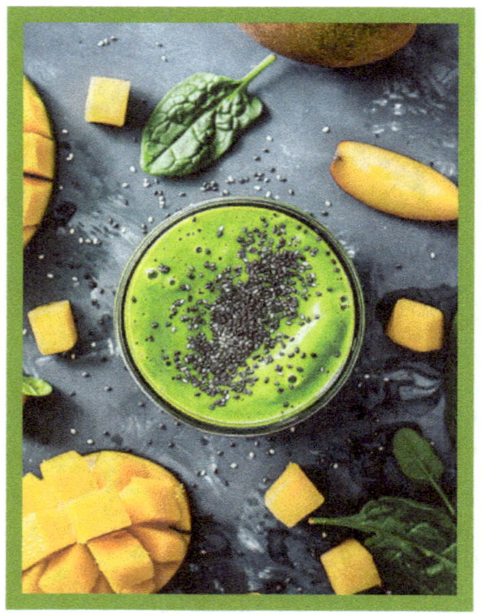

Benefits

Spinach is loaded with nutrients for skin, hair, and bone health.

Ingredients

1 cup pineapple chunks, 2 stalks of celery, 1/2 cucumber, 1/2 lime (juiced), 1 cup water

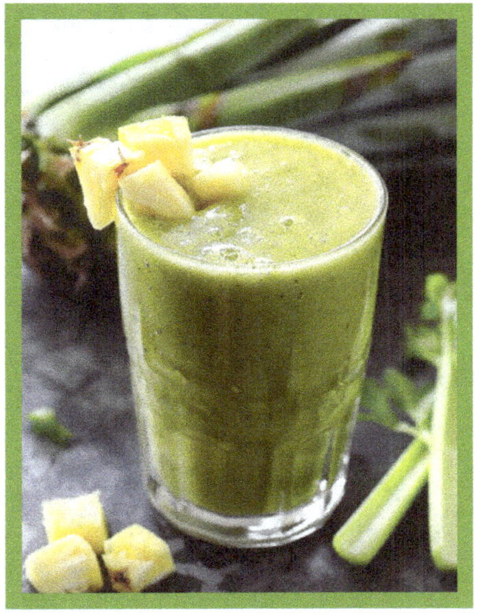

Benefits

Celery supports digestion and reduces inflammation.

Ingredients

1/2 cup cooked beets, 1/2 cup strawberries, 1/2 banana, 1 cup almond milk, 1 tsp cocoa powder

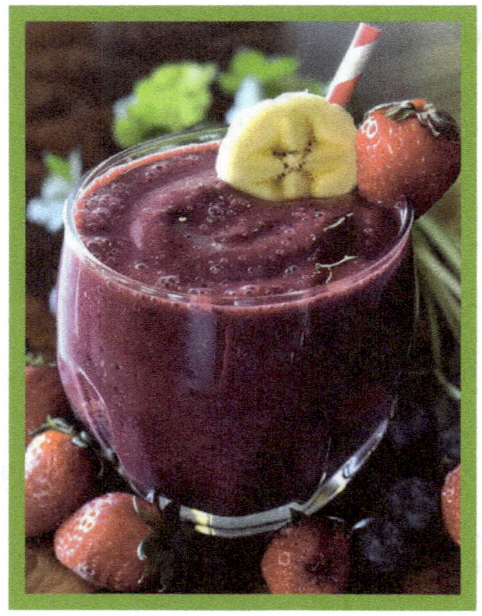

Benefits

Beets are great for cardiovascular health and reducing blood pressure.

Tropical Turmeric Twist

Ingredients

1/2 cup pineapple, 1/2 cup mango, 1/2 tsp turmeric powder, 1/2 lime (juiced), 1 cup coconut water

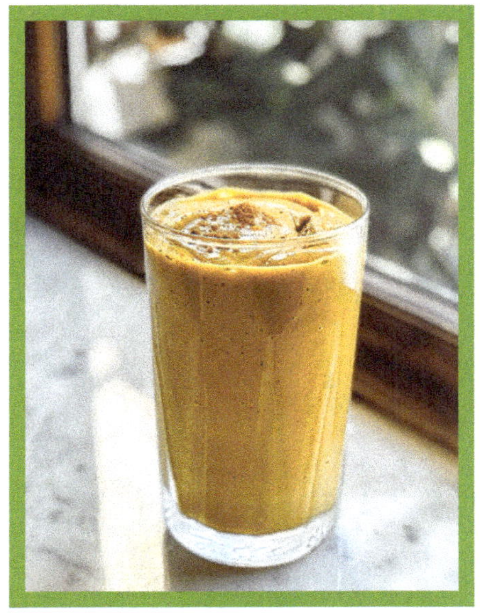

Benefits

Turmeric is a powerful anti-inflammatory and antioxidant.

Zingy Lemon Apple

Ingredients

1 green apple, 1/2 lemon (juiced), 1/2 inch fresh ginger, 1 cup spinach, 1 tsp honey, 1 cup water

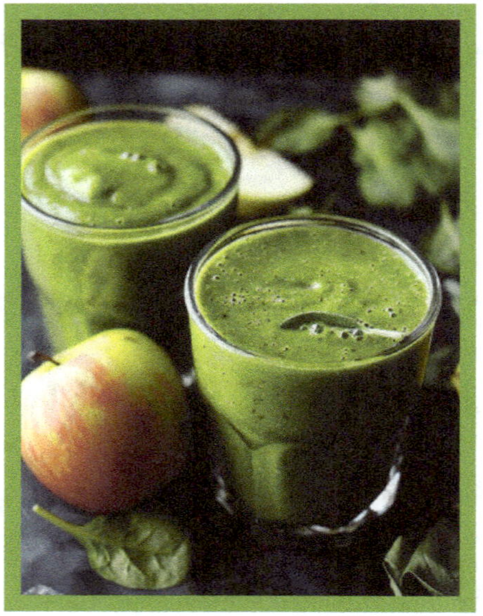

Benefits

Lemon juice detoxifies and alkalizes the body.

Ingredients

1 green apple, 1/2 inch ginger, 1 lemon, 1 cup spinach, 1/2 cucumber, 1 cup water

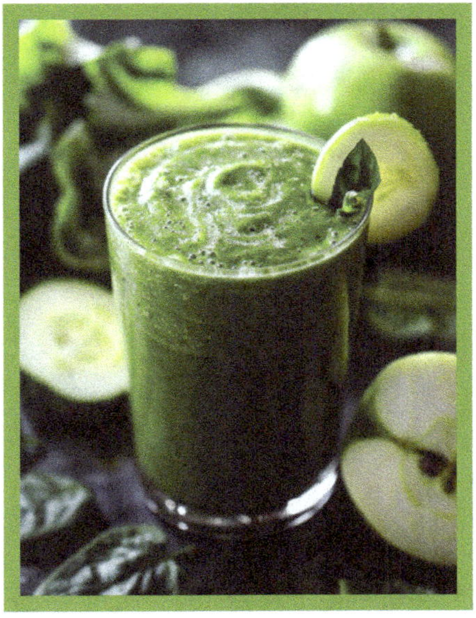

Benefits

Ginger aids digestion and has anti-inflammatory properties.

Tropical Charcoal Cleanse

Ingredients

1 cup pineapple, 1 banana, 1 tsp activated charcoal, 1 cup coconut water

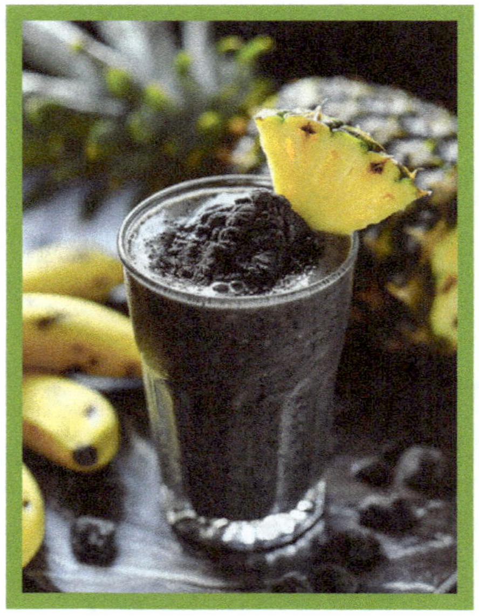

Benefits

Activated charcoal is known for trapping toxins for body removal.

Beet and Berry Liver Cleanse

Ingredients

1/2 beet, 1 cup mixed berries, 1/2 lemon, 1 tbsp flaxseed, 1 cup water

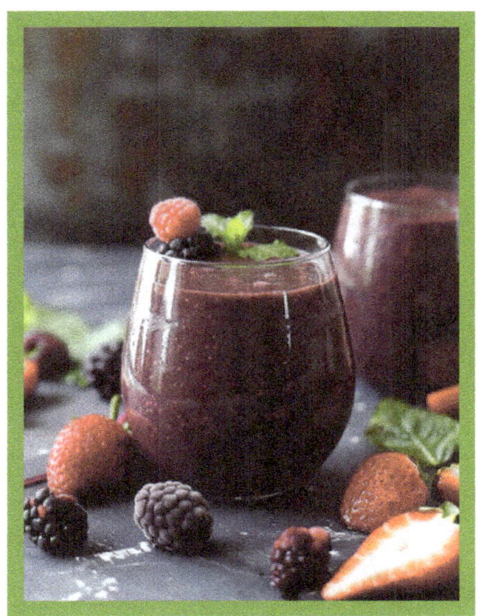

Benefits

Beets support liver detoxification and improve blood flow.

Cucumber Melon Hydrator

Ingredients

1 cup honeydew melon, 1/2 cucumber, 1/2 lime, mint leaves, 1 cup water

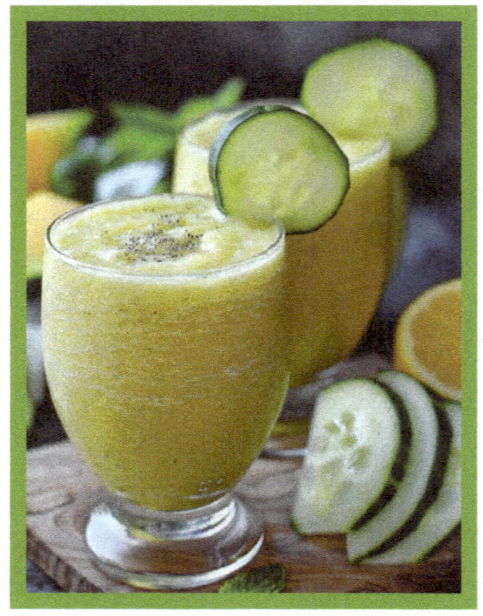

Benefits

Honeydew melon is hydrating and rich in vitamins and minerals.

Carrot Lemonade Flush

Ingredients

2 carrots, 1 apple, 1/2 lemon, 1 inch turmeric, 1 cup water

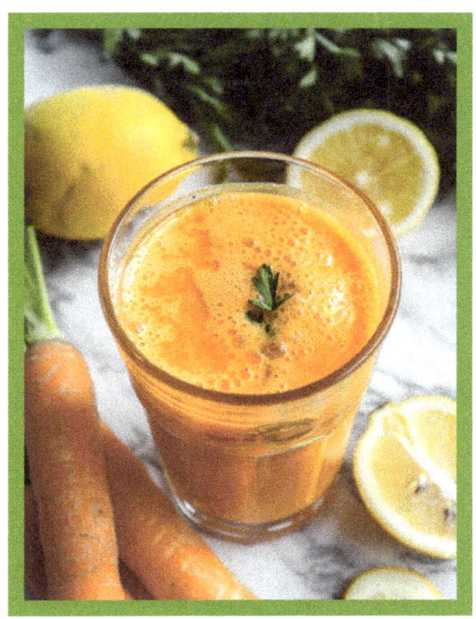

Benefits

Carrots are high in beta-carotene and fiber for digestive health.

Pineapple Kale Digestive

Ingredients

1 cup pineapple, 1 cup kale, 1/2 inch ginger, 1/2 avocado, 1 cup water

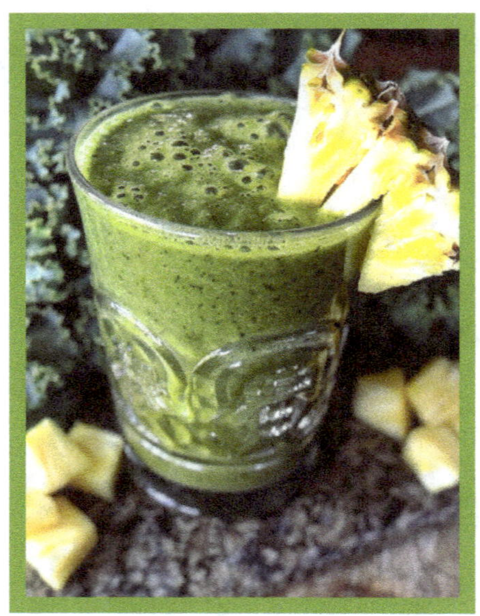

Benefits

Kale is nutrient-dense, supporting overall health and detoxification.

Spicy Watermelon Mint

Ingredients

2 cups watermelon, 1/2 lime, 1/4 tsp cayenne pepper, mint leaves, 1 cup water

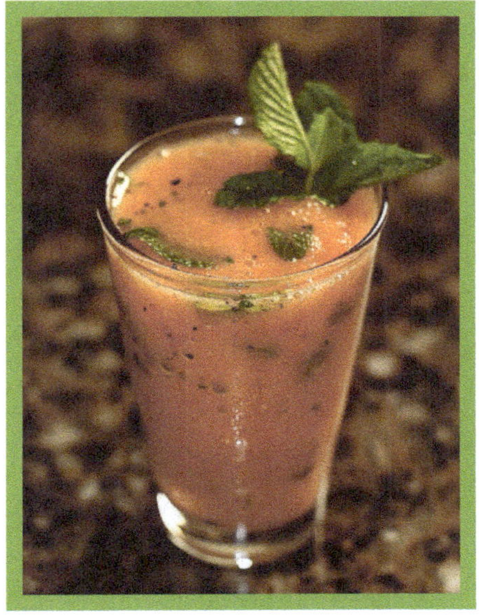

Benefits

Watermelon is great for hydration and the cayenne pepper boosts metabolism.

Sweet Potato Ginger Boost

Ingredients

1/2 cooked sweet potato, 1 carrot, 1/2 inch ginger, 1/2 apple, 1 cup almond milk

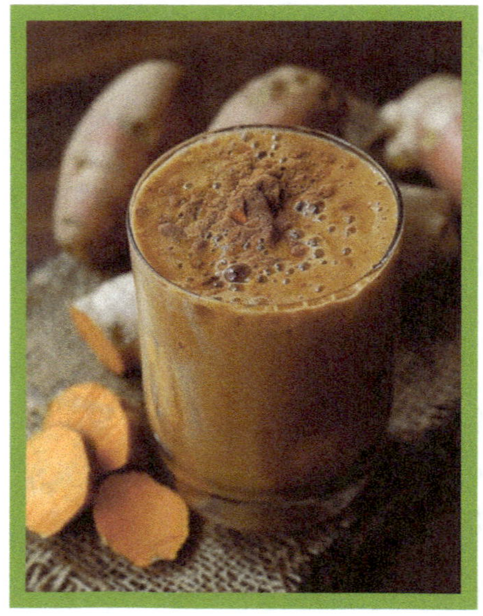

Benefits

Sweet potatoes are a good source of beta-carotene and vitamins.

Ingredients

1 cup blueberries, 1 banana, 1 tsp spirulina, 1 tbsp chia seeds, 1 cup almond milk

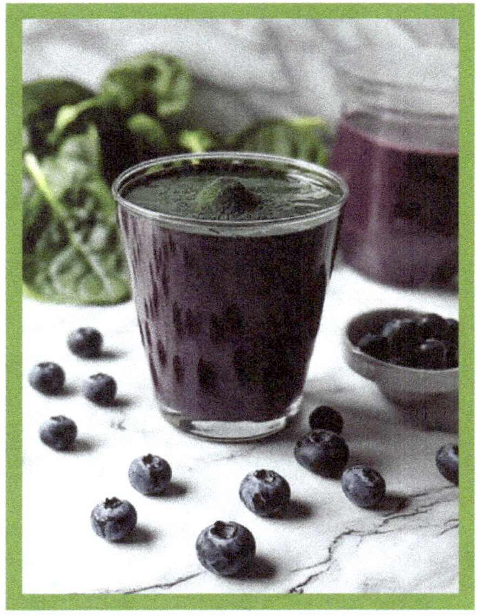

Benefits

Spirulina is a powerful antioxidant and source of vegan protein.

Avocado Kiwi Zen

Ingredients

1/2 avocado, 2 kiwis, 1/2 cucumber, 1 cup spinach, 1/2 lime, 1 cup water

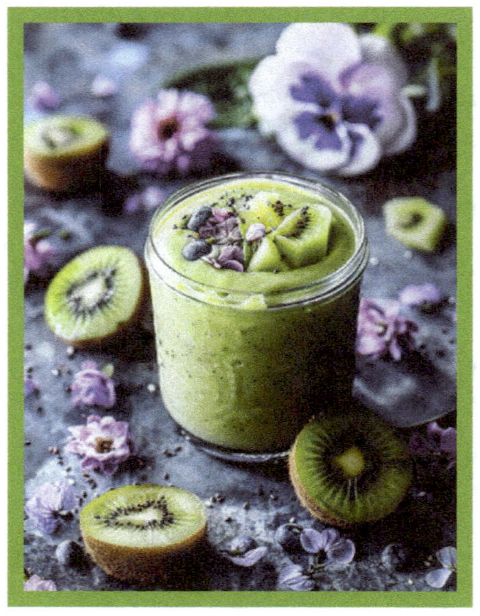

Benefits

Avocados provide healthy fats and fiber to keep you full longer.

Ingredients

1 orange, 1/2 grapefruit, 1/2 lemon, 1 inch turmeric, 1 cup water, a handful of ice

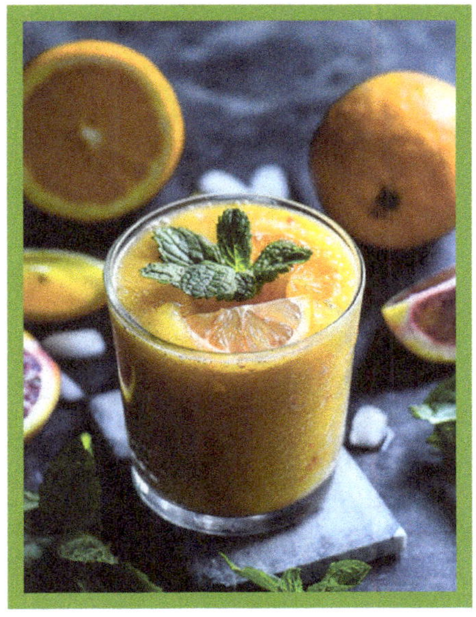

Benefits

Turmeric is known for its anti-inflammatory properties.

Vibrant Beet Cleanser

Ingredients

1 small beet, 1 apple, 1 carrot, 1 inch ginger, 1 cup water

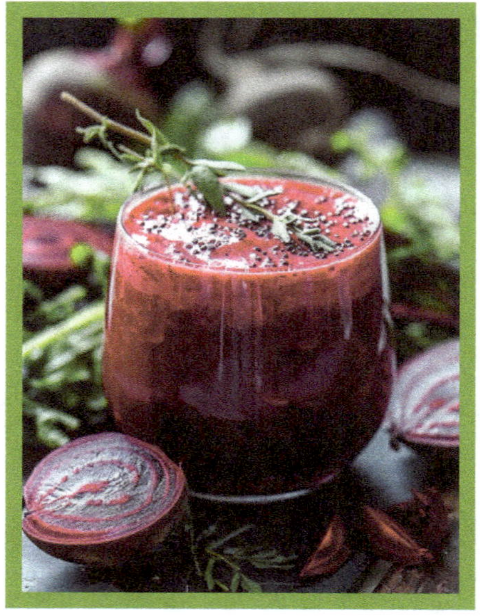

Benefits

Beets help cleanse the liver and improve blood quality.

Green Ginger Hydrator

Ingredients

1 cup spinach, 1/2 cucumber, 1/2 apple, 1 inch ginger, 1 tablespoon lemon juice, 1 cup coconut water

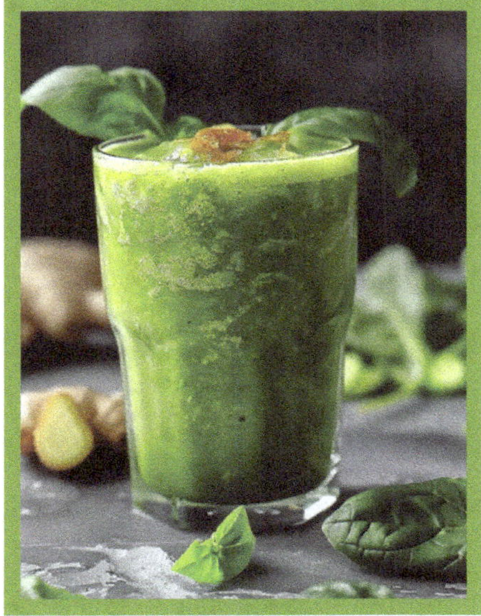

Benefits

Ginger aids in digestion and helps reduce inflammation.

Berry Flax Boost

Ingredients

1 cup mixed berries, 1 banana, 1 tablespoon flaxseed, 1 cup almond milk

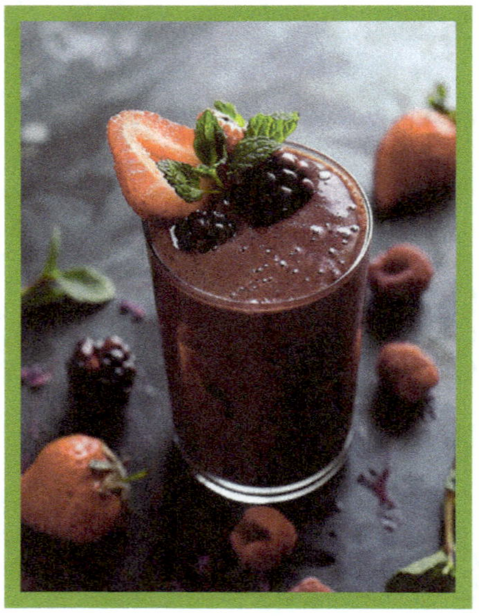

Benefits

Flaxseeds are rich in omega-3 fatty acids and fiber.

Tropical Turmeric Flush

Ingredients

1/2 cup pineapple, 1/2 cup mango, 1/2 teaspoon turmeric, 1/2 banana, 1 cup coconut water

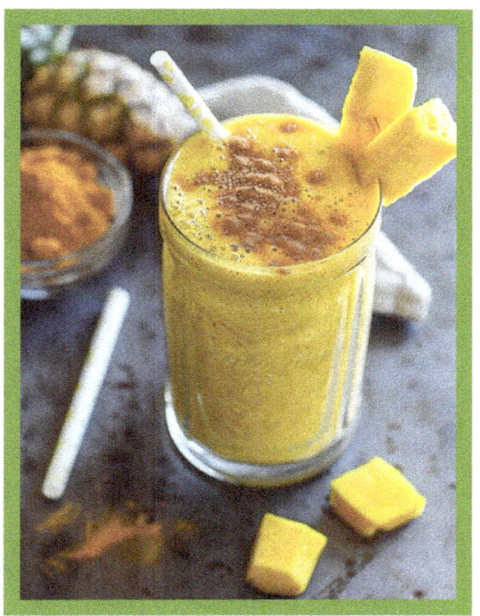

Benefits

Pineapple contains bromelain, an enzyme that aids digestion.

Cooling Cucumber Mint

Ingredients

1 cucumber, 1/2 cup mint leaves, 1 tablespoon lime juice, 1/2 green apple, 1 cup water

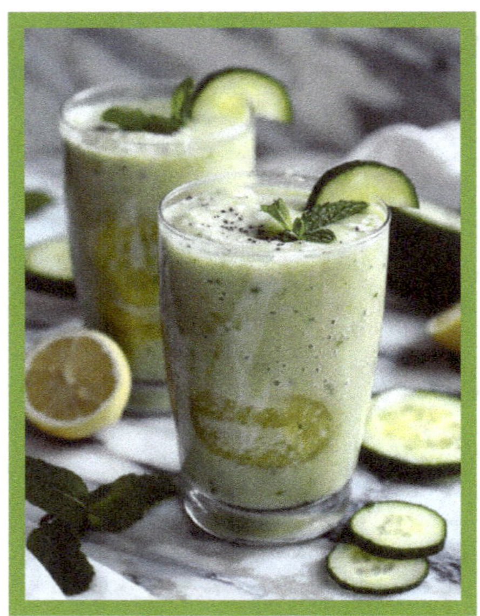

Benefits

Cucumber is highly hydrating and good for skin health.

Ingredients

1/2 avocado, 1 cup spinach, 1/2 banana, 1/2 orange, 1 cup water

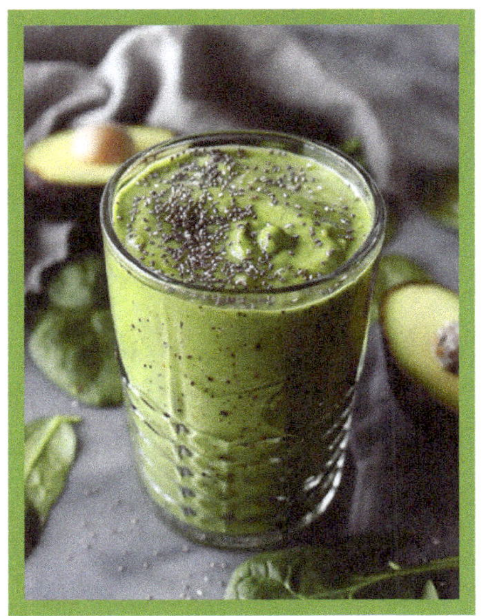

Benefits

Avocado offers healthy fats, promoting satiety and absorption of nutrients.

Carrot Apple Zinger

Ingredients

2 carrots, 1 apple, 1 inch ginger, 1 tablespoon lemon juice, 1 cup water

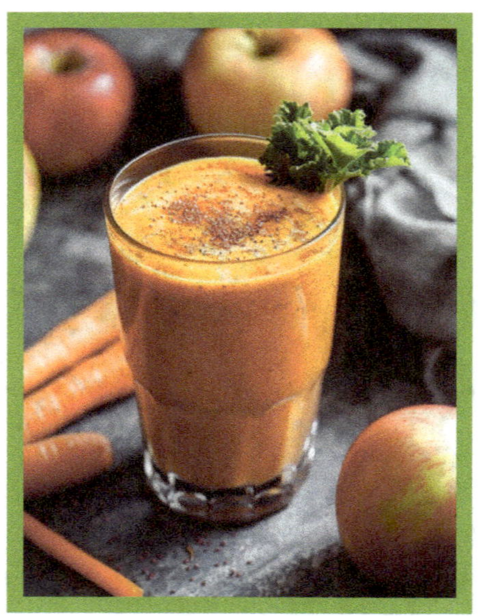

Benefits

Carrots are high in beta-carotene, essential for eye health.

Pomegranate Berry Blast

Ingredients

1/2 cup pomegranate seeds, 1/2 cup mixed berries, 1 banana, 1 cup spinach, 1 cup water

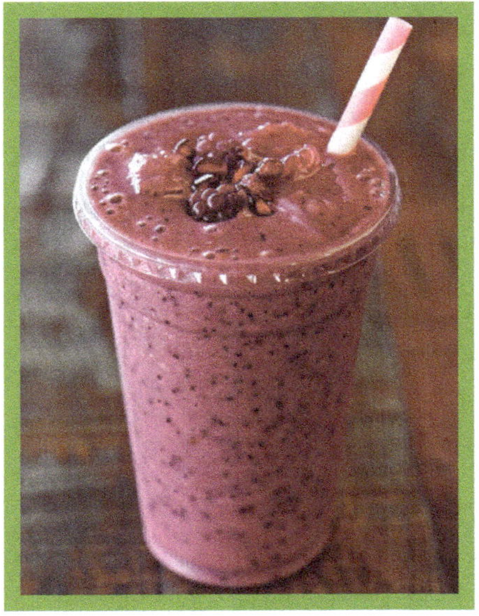

Benefits

Pomegranate is packed with antioxidants for heart health.

Kiwi Lime Refresh

Ingredients

2 kiwis, juice of 1 lime, 1/2 cucumber, 1 cup spinach, 1 cup water

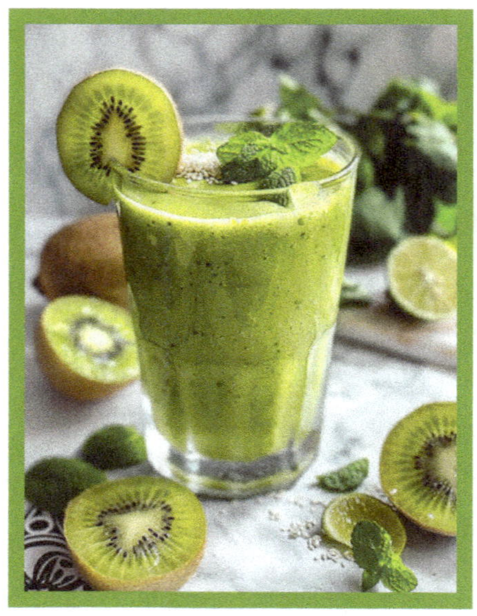

Benefits

Kiwi is rich in vitamin C, boosting the immune system.

Ultimate Green Detox

Ingredients

1 cup kale, 1/2 cup spinach, 1 green apple, 1/2 cucumber, 1 tablespoon parsley, 1 cup coconut water

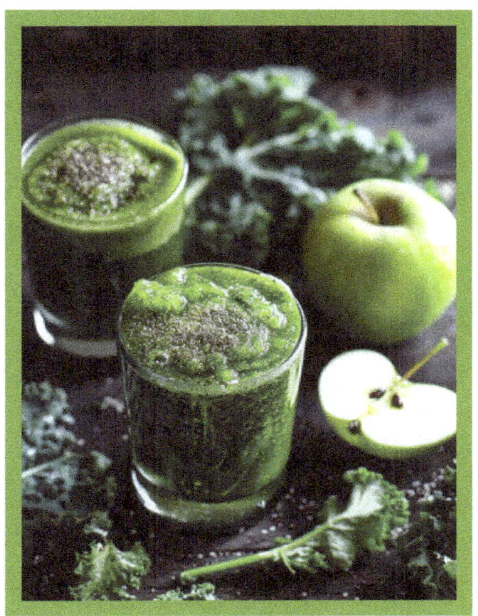

Benefits

Kale is a nutrient powerhouse, packed with vitamins A, K, and C.

Berry Beet Reviver

Ingredients

1/2 cup cooked beet, 1 cup mixed berries, 1 banana, 1 tablespoon flaxseed oil, 1 cup almond milk

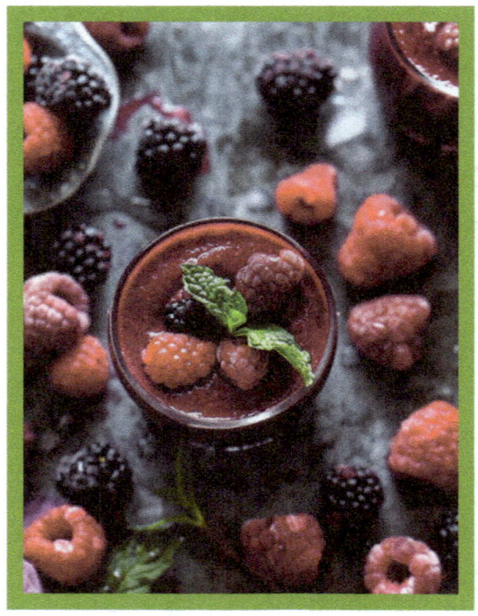

Benefits

Beets detoxify the liver and improve blood flow.

Ginger Turmeric Tonic

Ingredients

1 inch ginger, 1/2 teaspoon turmeric, 1 carrot, 1 orange, 1 cup pineapple, 1 cup water

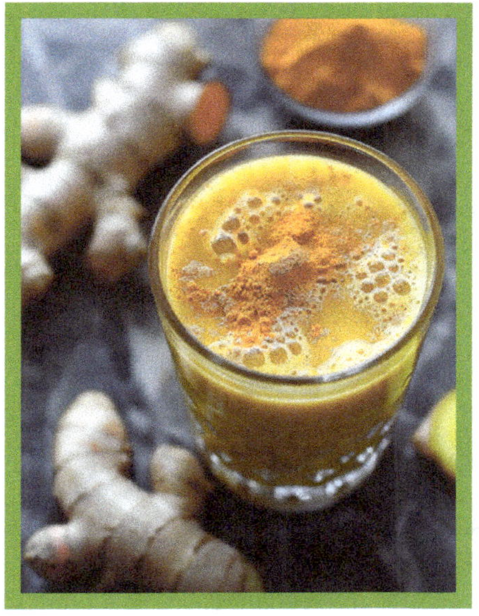

Benefits

Turmeric and ginger offer anti-inflammatory and digestive benefits.

Citrus Flush Smoothie

Ingredients

1 grapefruit, 1 orange, 1 lemon (juiced), 1 cup spinach,
1 tablespoon chia seeds, 1 cup water

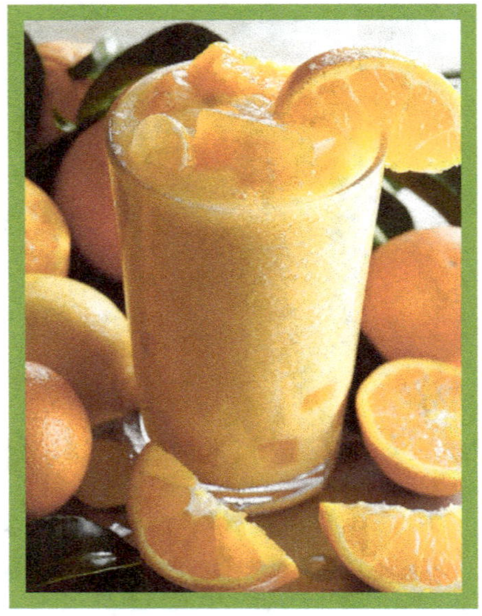

Benefits

Citrus fruits are rich in vitamin C, boosting the
immune system.

Ingredients

1 cup pineapple, 1/2 cucumber, 1/2 lime (juiced), 1 cup kale, 1 tablespoon mint, 1 cup water

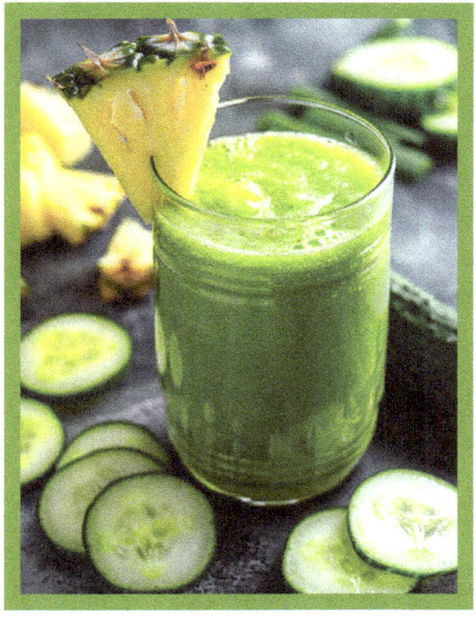

Benefits

Pineapple contains bromelain, aiding digestion and inflammation.

Ingredients

1/2 avocado, 1/2 banana, 1 cup spinach, 1/2 apple, 1 tablespoon lemon juice, 1 cup almond milk

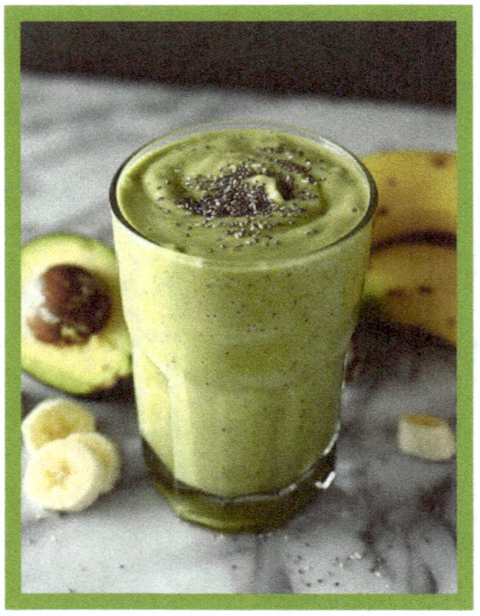

Benefits

Avocado provides healthy fats for energy and nutrient absorption.

Sweet Spirulina Boost

Ingredients

1 banana, 1 tablespoon spirulina powder, 1 cup spinach, 1/2 cup blueberries, 1 cup coconut water

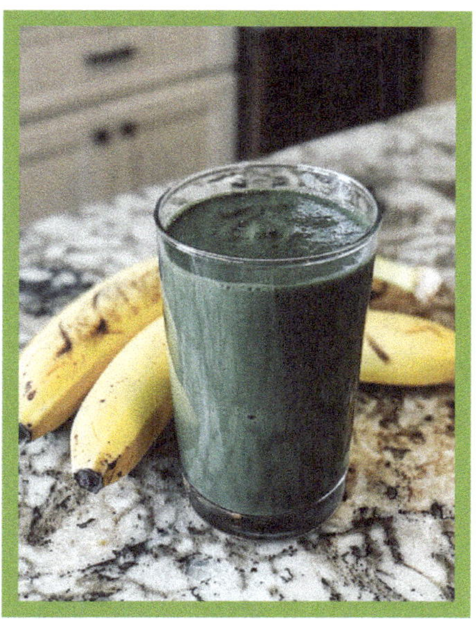

Benefits

Spirulina is a superfood rich in protein and antioxidants.

Ingredients

2 cups watermelon, 1/2 cucumber, 1 cup mint leaves, 1 cup water, juice of 1 lime

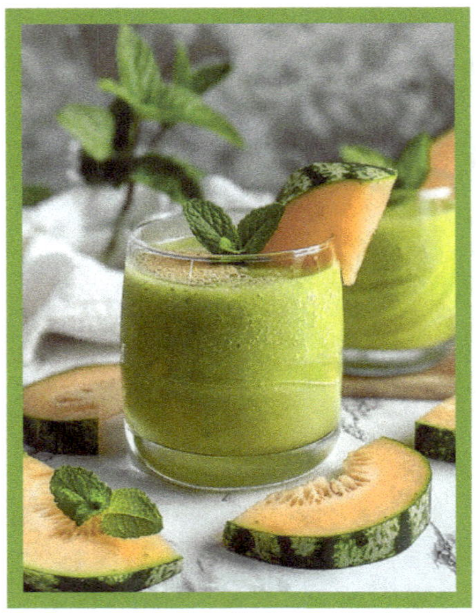

Benefits

Watermelon is hydrating and helps flush out toxins.

Carrot Ginger Flush

Ingredients

2 carrots, 1 inch ginger, 1 apple, juice of 1/2 lemon, 1 cup water

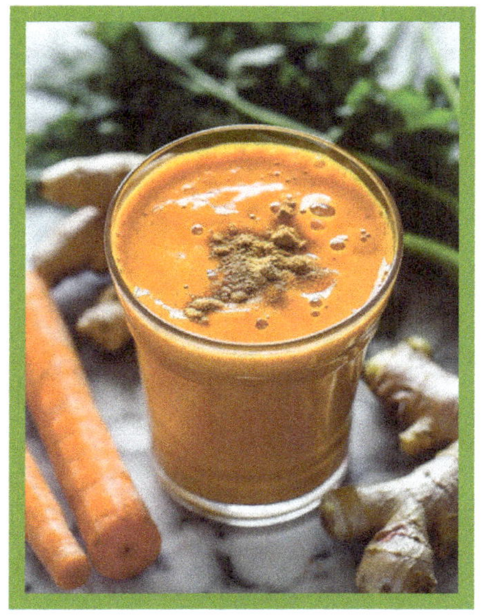

Benefits

Carrots are rich in beta-carotene, vital for vision and skin health.

Zesty Lime Detox

Ingredients

1/2 lime (juiced), 1 kiwi, 1/2 cucumber, 1 cup spinach, 1 green apple, 1 cup water

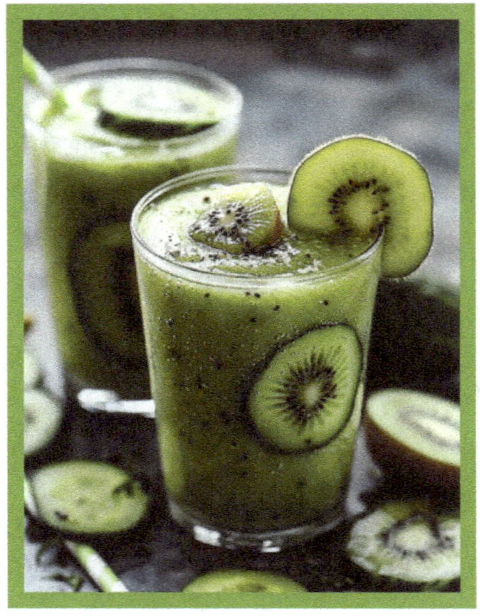

Benefits

Lime is detoxifying and adds a refreshing zest.

Ingredients

2 stalks of celery, 1/2 green apple, 1/2 banana, 1 cup spinach, 1 tablespoon lemon juice, 1 cup water

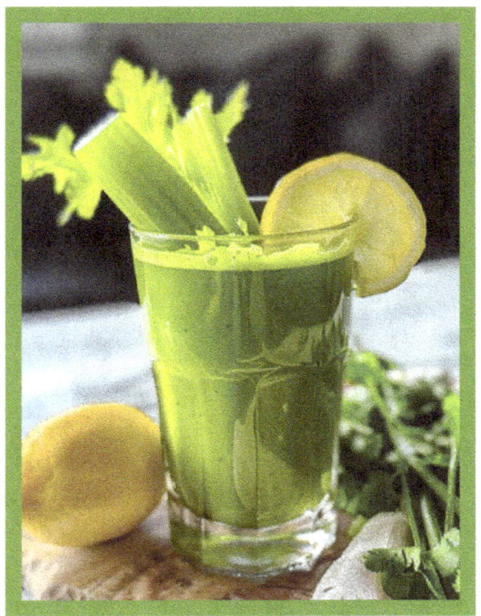

Benefits

Celery aids in hydration and reduces inflammation.

Golden Mango Detox

Ingredients

1 cup mango, 1/2 teaspoon turmeric, 1/2 banana, 1/2 orange, 1 tablespoon flax seeds, 1 cup almond milk

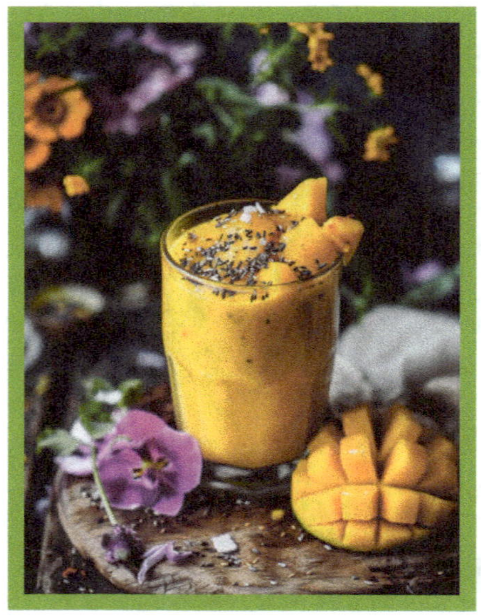

Benefits

Turmeric is a powerful anti-inflammatory and antioxidant.

Berry Spinach Cleanse

Ingredients

1 cup mixed berries (strawberries, blueberries, raspberries), 1 cup spinach, 1 tablespoon chia seeds, 1 cup coconut water

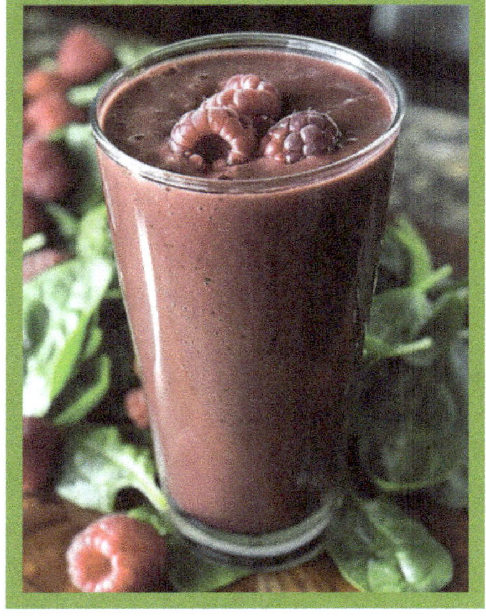

Benefits

Berries are rich in antioxidants which support detoxification.

Ingredients

1 pear, 1 inch piece of ginger, 1/2 lemon (juiced), 1 cup kale, 1 tablespoon honey, 1 cup water

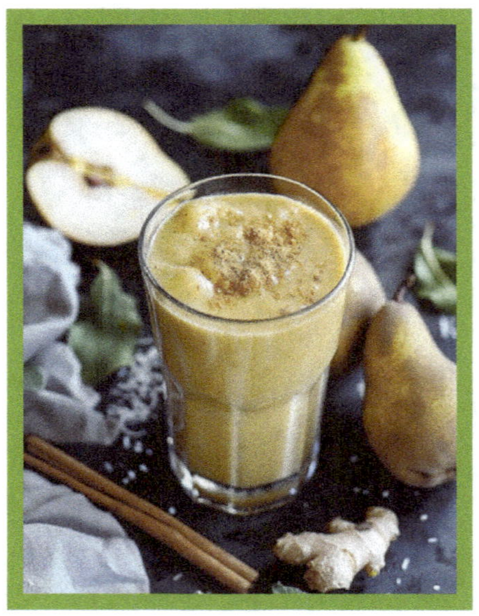

Benefits

Ginger stimulates digestion and boosts metabolism.

Refreshing Cucumber Mint

Ingredients

1 cucumber, 1/2 cup fresh mint leaves, 1/2 lime (juiced), 1/2 green apple, 1 cup water

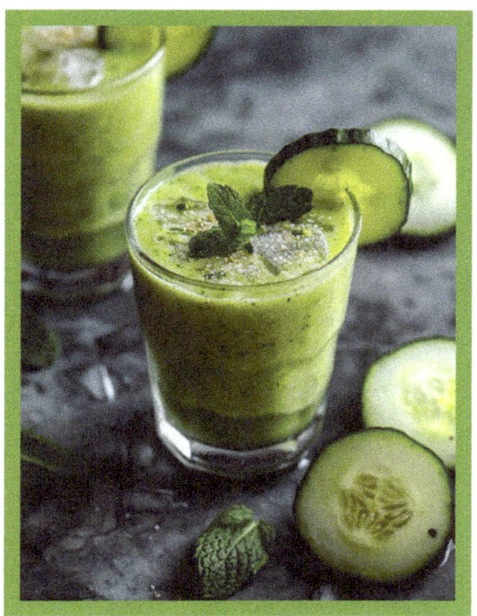

Benefits

Mint promotes digestion and soothes the stomach.

Tropical Green Energy

Ingredients

1 cup pineapple, 1/2 banana, 1 cup kale, 1/2 avocado, 1 tablespoon spirulina, 1 cup coconut water

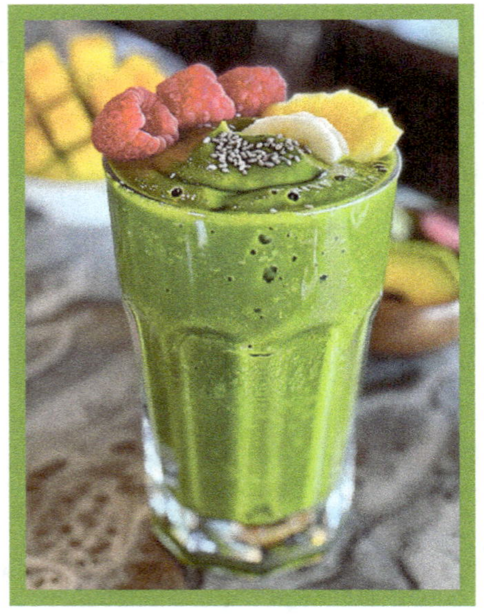

Benefits

Spirulina is a nutrient-dense algae that boosts energy and vitality.

Beetroot Ginger Bliss

Ingredients

1 small beetroot, 1 apple, 1 inch ginger, 1/2 lemon (juiced), 1 cup water

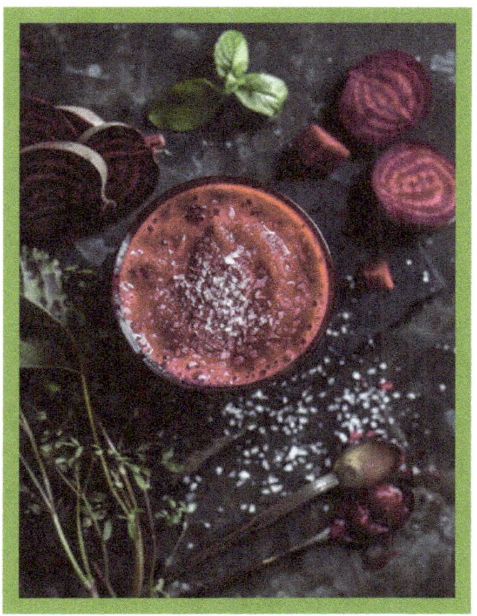

Benefits

Beetroot helps purify the blood and liver.

Carrot Apple Ginger

Ingredients

2 carrots, 1 green apple, 1 inch ginger, 1/2 lemon (juiced), 1 cup water

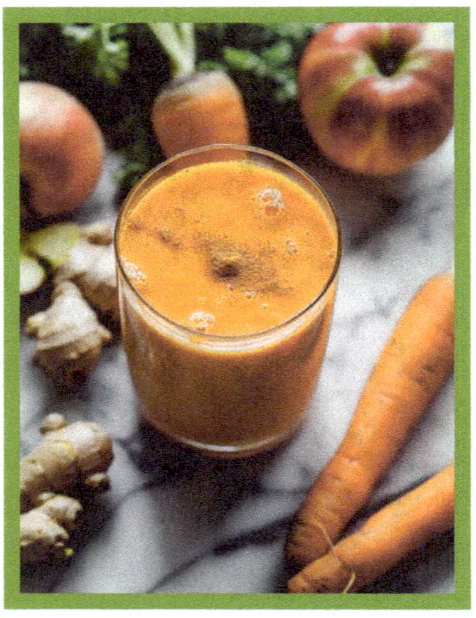

Benefits

Carrots are high in vitamin A, supporting eye health and skin.

Zingy Lemonade Detox

Ingredients

1 lemon (juiced), 1/2 cucumber, 1 tablespoon maple syrup, 1 cup water, a pinch of cayenne pepper

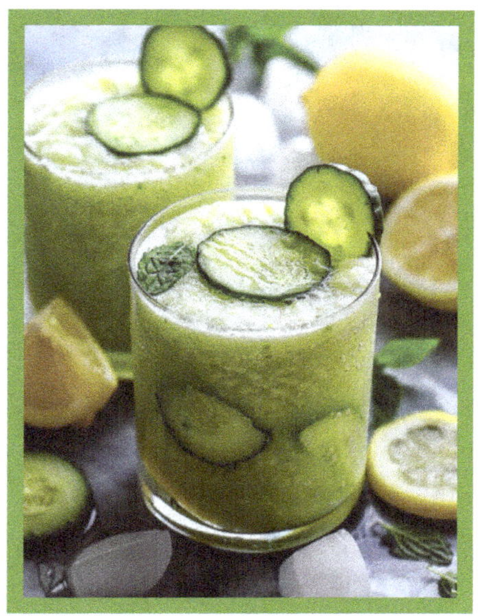

Benefits

Lemon juice aids in detoxification and digestion.

Avocado Berry Smoothie

Ingredients

1/2 avocado, 1 cup mixed berries, 1/2 banana, 1 cup spinach, 1 cup almond milk

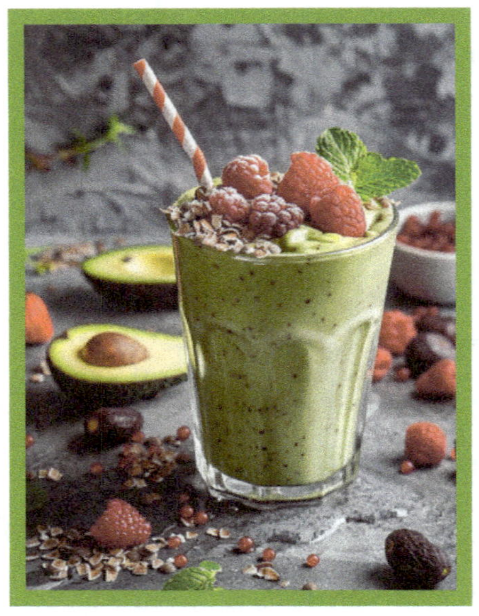

Benefits

Avocado adds creaminess and provides healthy fats and fiber.

Lemon Ginger Zest

Ingredients

1 lemon (juiced), 1 inch ginger, 1 apple, 1 cup spinach, 1/2 cucumber, 1 cup water

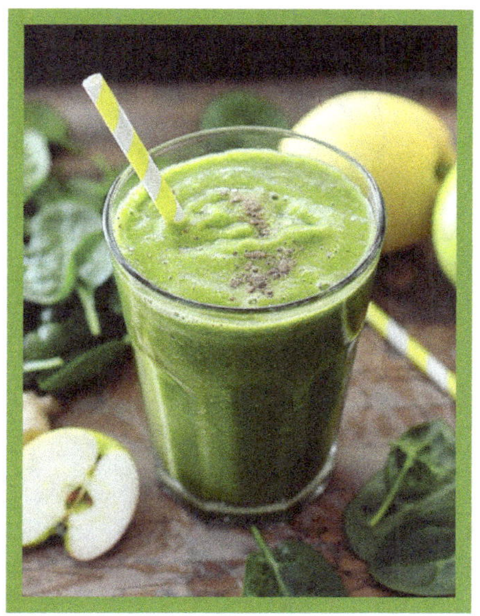

Benefits

Ginger promotes digestion and has anti-inflammatory properties.

Turmeric Sunrise

Ingredients

1/2 cup pineapple, 1 banana, 1/2 teaspoon turmeric, 1/2 cup mango, 1 cup orange juice

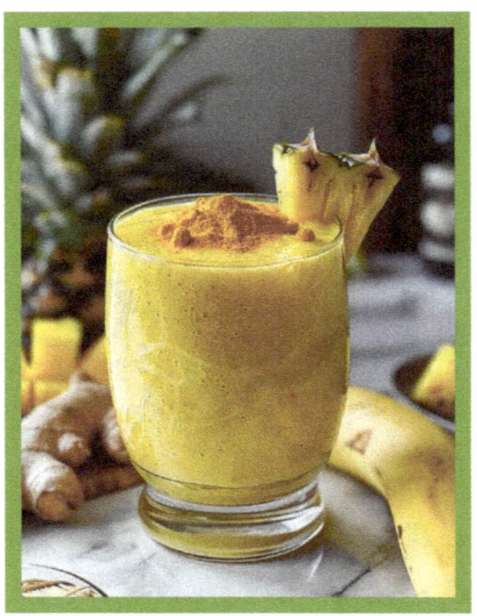

Benefits

Turmeric is known for its antioxidant and anti-inflammatory effects.

Ingredients

1 cup brewed green tea (cooled), 1 cup kale, 1/2 apple, 1/2 banana, 1 teaspoon honey

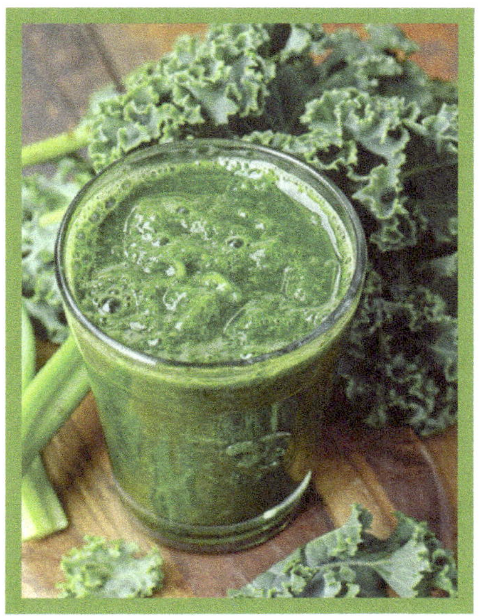

Benefits

Green tea enhances fat burning and improves brain function.

Beetroot and Berry

Ingredients

1 small beetroot, 1 cup mixed berries, 1 orange, 1/2 banana, 1 cup water

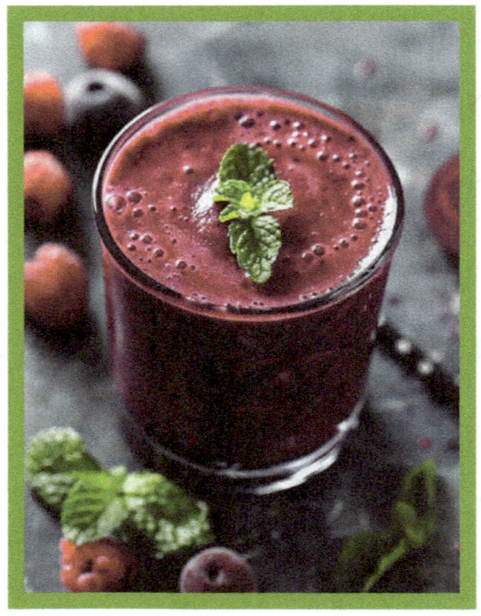

Benefits

Beetroot helps lower blood pressure and boost exercise performance.

Cucumber Kiwi Cleanse

Ingredients

1 cucumber, 2 kiwis, 1/2 lemon (juiced), 1 cup water, handful of mint

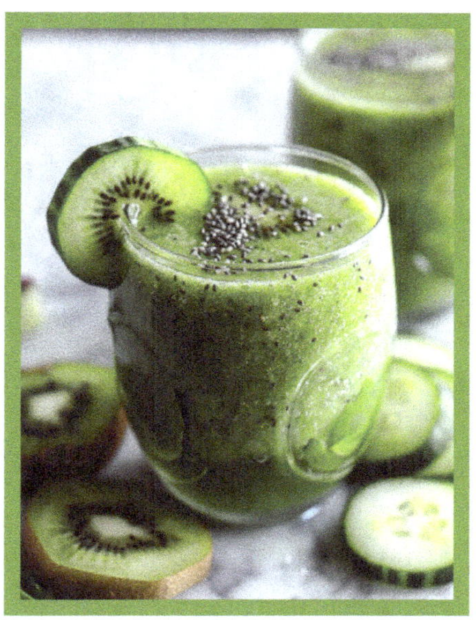

Benefits

Kiwi is high in Vitamin C and dietary fiber for improved digestion and immunity.

Spicy Avocado Kick

Ingredients

1/2 avocado, 1/2 teaspoon cayenne pepper, 1 cup
spinach, 1/2 lime (juiced), 1 cup almond milk

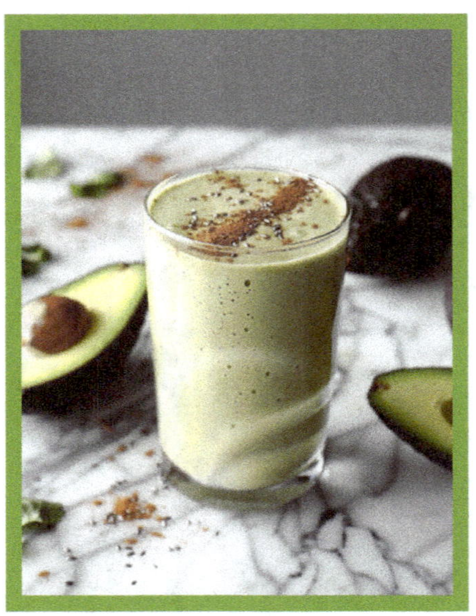

Benefits

Cayenne pepper boosts metabolism and aids in
digestion.

Pineapple Celery Splash

Ingredients

1 cup pineapple, 2 stalks celery, 1/2 cucumber, 1/2 cup parsley, 1 cup coconut water

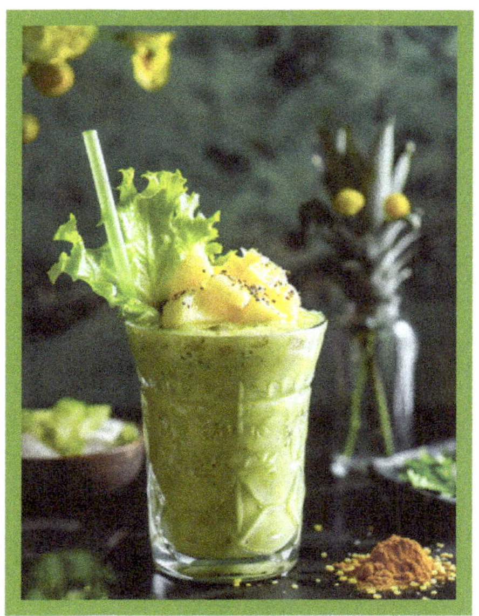

Benefits

Celery supports hydration and reduces inflammation.

Sweet Spinach Revival

Ingredients

1 cup spinach, 1/2 apple, 1/2 banana, 1 tablespoon almond butter, 1 cup almond milk

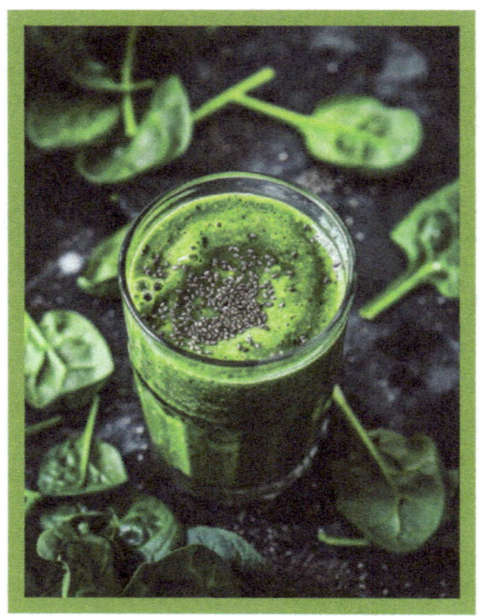

Benefits

Spinach is packed with nutrients for energy and detoxification.

Carrot Lemon Boost

Ingredients

2 carrots, juice of 1 lemon, 1 inch turmeric, 1 cup water, 1 apple

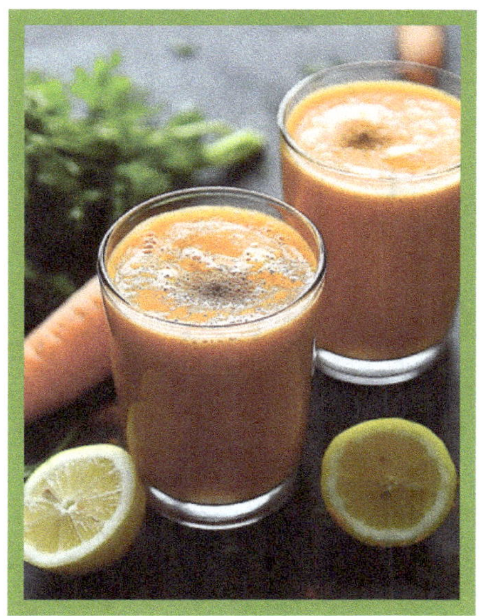

Benefits

Carrots are rich in beta-carotene and fiber, promoting eye health and digestion.

Berry Flax Fusion

Ingredients

1 cup mixed berries (strawberries, blueberries, raspberries), 1 banana, 2 tablespoons flaxseeds, 1 cup water

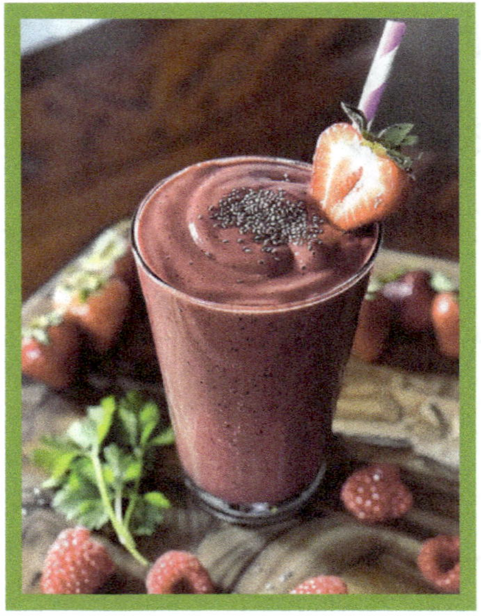

Benefits

Flaxseeds are high in omega-3 fatty acids and fiber for detoxification and heart health.

Refreshing Mint Melon

Ingredients

2 cups watermelon, 1 cucumber, 1/2 cup mint leaves, 1 lime (juiced), 1 cup water

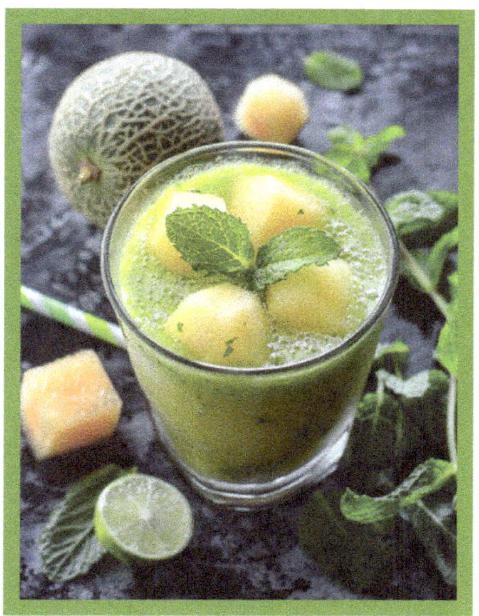

Benefits

Watermelon is hydrating and helps flush toxins from the body.

Golden Glow Smoothie

Ingredients

1/2 cup pineapple, 1 carrot, 1/2 teaspoon turmeric, 1 orange, 1 cup water

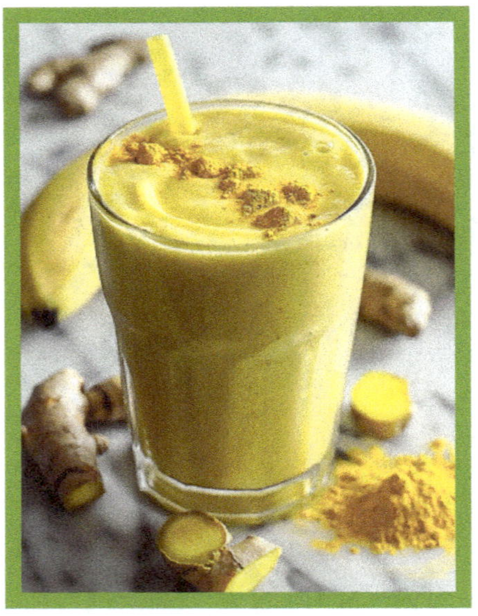

Benefits

Turmeric offers anti-inflammatory and antioxidant benefits.

Green Detox Twist

Ingredients

1 cup spinach, 1/2 green apple, 1/2 lemon (juiced), 1 inch ginger, 1 cucumber, 1 cup water

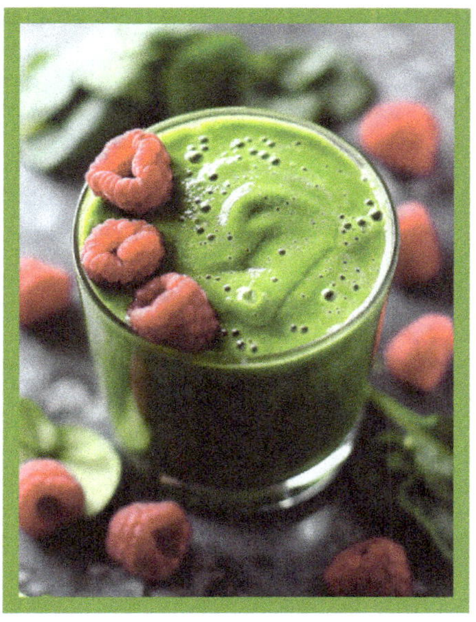

Benefits

Spinach is rich in chlorophyll, which supports detoxification.

Ingredients

1 small beet, 1 cup mixed berries, 1 banana, 1 tablespoon chia seeds, 1 cup almond milk

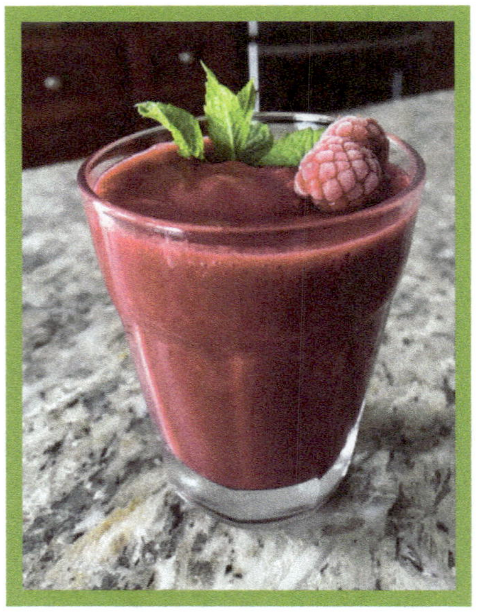

Benefits

Beets cleanse the liver and improve blood flow.

Spicy Pineapple Cleanse

Ingredients

1 cup pineapple, 1/2 teaspoon cayenne pepper, 1 carrot, 1/2 lime (juiced), 1 cup water

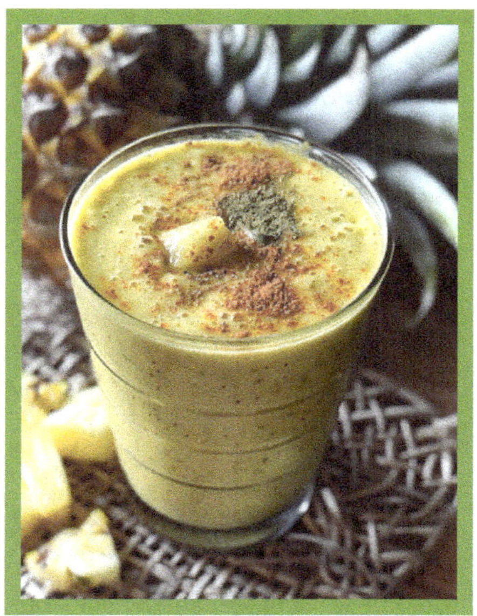

Benefits

Cayenne pepper boosts metabolism and aids in digestion.

Ingredients

1/2 avocado, 1/2 banana, 1 cup spinach, 1/2 cucumber, 1 cup almond milk, 1 tablespoon lime juice

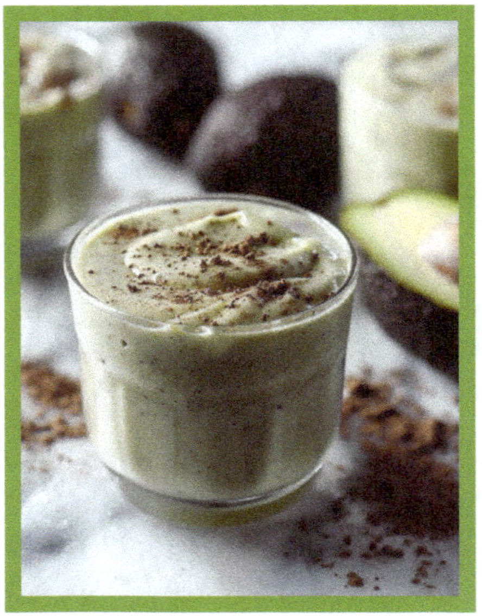

Benefits

Avocado is loaded with heart-healthy monounsaturated fatty acids.

Ingredients

1 green apple, 2 stalks celery, 1 inch ginger, 1/2 lemon (juiced), 1 cup water

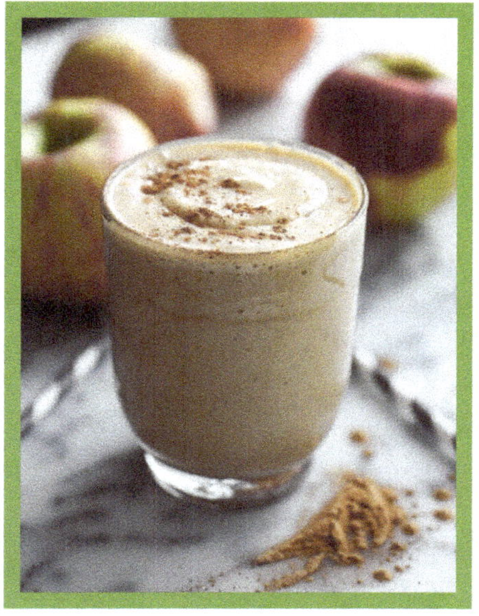

Benefits

Celery acts as a diuretic, supporting kidney function.

Tropical Turmeric Flush

Ingredients

1/2 cup mango, 1/2 cup pineapple, 1/2 teaspoon turmeric, 1/2 banana, 1 cup coconut water

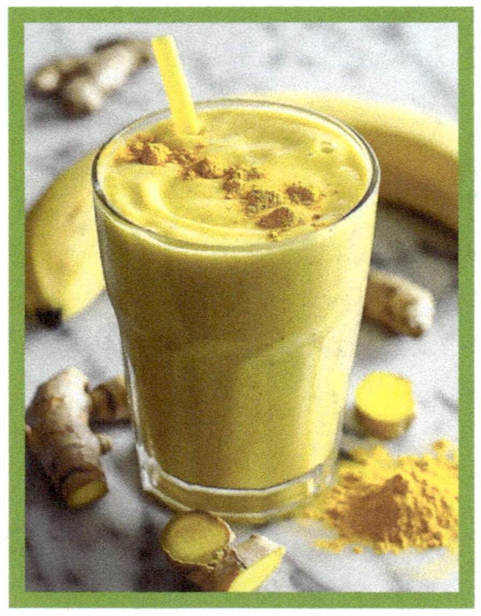

Benefits

Mango is full of fiber and vitamins, promoting a healthy gut.

Kiwi Cucumber Slush

Ingredients

2 kiwis, 1 cucumber, 1/2 cup spinach, 1/2 apple, 1 cup water

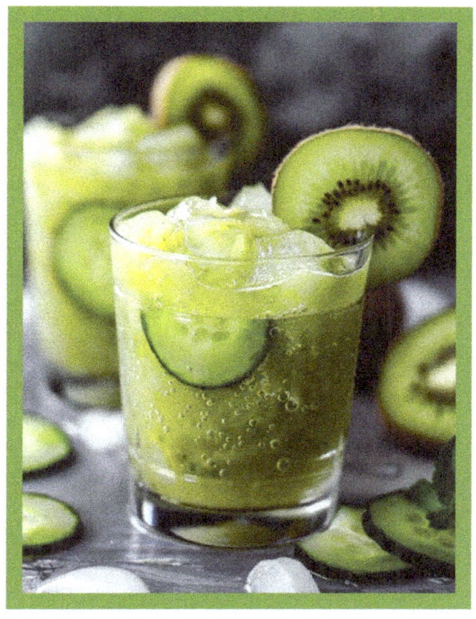

Benefits

Kiwi is an excellent source of Vitamin C and aids in digestion.

9 798322 539964